Image-Guided Radiation Therapy in Lymphoma Management

Image-Guided Radiation Therapy in Lymphoma Management:

The Increasing Role of Functional Imaging

edited by:

Roger M Macklis, MD

*Department of Radiation Oncology and
Taussig Cancer Center,
Cleveland Clinic Lerner College of Medicine,
Cleveland, Ohio, USA*

Peter S Conti, MD, PhD

*Professor of Radiology, Pharmacy and
Biomedical Engineering,
University of Southern California,
Los Angeles, California, USA*

Chief Editorial Assistant:

Nidhi Sharma, MD
*Clinical Fellow,
Department of Diagnostic Radiology,
Cleveland Clinic,
Cleveland, Ohio, USA*

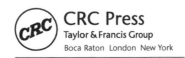

CRC Press
Taylor & Francis Group
Boca Raton London New York

CRC Press is an imprint of the
Taylor & Francis Group, an **informa** business

CRC Press
Taylor & Francis Group
6000 Broken Sound Parkway NW, Suite 300
Boca Raton, FL 33487-2742

First issued in paperback 2019

© 2010 by Taylor & Francis Group, LLC
CRC Press is an imprint of Taylor & Francis Group, an Informa business

No claim to original U.S. Government works

ISBN-13: 978-1-4200-5874-1 (hbk)
ISBN-13: 978-0-367-38448-7 (pbk)

A CIP record for this book is available from the British Library.
Library of Congress Cataloging-in-Publication Data

Typeset by Amnet International, Dublin, Ireland

Visit the Taylor & Francis Web site at
http://www.taylorandfrancis.com

and the CRC Press Web site at
http://www.crcpress.com

Dedication

For my two sons Andrew and Paul, who constantly push me to improve my abilities in computer technology and image manipulation. Some day I hope to approach their levels of technical sophistication. – Roger M Macklis

To my wife and family for their continuing support, love and encouragement – Peter S Conti

To my parents and my husband Ankit, for their belief in me and constant inspiration to achieve greater heights. – Nidhi Sharma.

Table of contents

Preface

Image-Guided Radiation Therapy (IGRT) can be seen as the latest step in the evolution of radiation therapy from a loosely focused directional therapeutic to a more tightly focused highly targeted biologically active form of treatment for cancer. As the degree of targeting increases, there is concomitant reduction of non-target or "innocent bystander" damage to normal tissue within the treatment site. Refining the target and differentiating it from nearby normal structures are key factors in driving current interest in IGRT and its potential for reducing normal tissue damage.

An important component of risk minimization involves developing algorithms to guide the direction of delivered dose to the location of clonogenically viable target cells. This location will usually include areas of visible tumor and radiographically detectable marginal cancer masses but usually also involves a more poorly defined region in which tumor cell density may be too low to detect with conventional radiographic studies. Advanced anatomic imaging procedures, such as CT, MRI, and ultrasound, have been readily incorporated into the armamentarium of the radiation oncologist and the treatment planning team. For some tumor types, volumetric imaging obtained from these modalities provides sufficient information for successful treatment, while in other cases, more sophisticated approaches, such as use of cone-beam CT, are necessary.

For malignant lymphoma, the task of precision targeting can be more elusive, as tumor boundaries are not always well demarcated anatomically. In the case of lymphoma, PET (positron emission tomography) imaging with the radiotracer ^{18}F-Fluorodeoxyglucose (^{18}FDG) to image tumor glucose utilization has proven particularly rewarding in staging as well as monitor the effects of treatment. PET essentially allows real-time in vivo observation of clinically relevant biological processes taking place within normal and transformed tissue. While compounds such as ^{18}FDG have been shown to be useful as tumor markers and staging indicators, new families of radiotracers are now being evaluated as potential indicators of tumor responsiveness and surrogate clinical tumor control endpoints in management of malignant lymphoma. Serial changes in the pattern observed with ^{18}FDG-PET studies of patients undergoing chemotherapy or radiation appear capable of predicting ultimate responses after a "trial" course of initial therapy. This serial imaging should in theory allow ineffective agents and treatments to be terminated and replaced with alternative treatment before serious toxicity or gross disease progression becomes manifest.

The application of these principles to clinical cancer medicine is now being formalized via comprehensive clinical trials and expert consensus reviews. This area remains very much a work in progress. In this manual, we have attempted to provide current highlights of the way that many different teams of experienced radiation oncologists and nuclear medicine physicians are using the new technologies of radiotherapy image guidance and correlated functional imaging. Each chapter is meant to be a summary of relevant clinical data and approaches to tumor control. An introductory chapter summarizes the way that image guidance and functional imaging are being applied to the problems of tumor control. These technologies are expanding very rapidly and it is likely that subsequent editions will require major rewriting as these technologies become more standardized. The manual is not meant to be encyclopedic in its coverage and will not take the place of more standard textbooks of radiation medicine. It should, however, serve as a starting point for students and practitioners interested in understanding the direction of this field.

At present true image guidance is still used in a minority of clinical radiation medicine protocols but the proportion is growing rapidly. Many expert radiation oncologists believe that ultimately nearly all therapeutic radiation exposures will be delivered using some form of image guidance. However we must avoid the tendency to use high technology for worthless levels of precision. IGRT will have to show its merits through comparative effectiveness studies conducted and graded by financially disinterested parties. The demonstration of the power of functional imaging in lymphoma management is already fulfilling this mandate and its application to highly conformal beam targeting will have to meet these same hurdles in order to convince skeptics of its ultimate worth.

The teams of authors responsible for writing and editing these chapters include nuclear medicine physicians, medical oncologists, and physicists, in addition to radiation oncologists. It is only through the recruitment and organization of such multidisciplinary teams that the optimal use of these technologies will ever be elucidated and brought to bear on clinical oncology. The use of IGRT and functional imaging are ideally suited for the management of some clinical situations, and it will be incumbent on current and future teams of multi-specialty physicians to identify exactly which groups of patients may be best served through this technologic application of carefully targeted treatment. One size will not fit all, and our decision to publish this introductory manual was meant to mark the beginning of an exciting technologic and medical journey that will lead to personalized care for patients suffering from this disease.

A century ago, radiation therapy was one of the only clinical treatments capable of producing true cure in malignant lymphoma patients. As cytotoxic chemotherapy became more widely available the dependence on radiotherapy diminished and it is currently much more rarely used in definitive therapy. It is possible that some of the principles and practices outlined in this volume will help build on a techno-biologic paradigm shift that may once again lead to a renaissance in the use of radiation medicine as a component of multimodality lymphoma management.

Contributors

Samuel T Chao Cleveland Clinic Foundation, Dept. of Radiation Oncology, Cleveland, Ohio, USA

Peter S Conti Biomedical Engineering and Pharmacy, University of Southern California, Los Angeles, California, USA

Angelika Bischof Delaloye University Hospital and University of Lausanne, Lausanne, Switzerland

Henry Blair Department of Radiation Oncology, Cleveland Clinic, Cleveland, Ohio, USA

Dominique Delbeke Department of Radiology and Radiological Sciences, Vanderbilt University Medical Center, Nashville, Tennessee, USA

Tony Y Eng Department of Radiation Oncology, University of Texas Health Science Center at San Antonio, and The Cancer Therapy and Research Center, San Antonio, Texas, USA

Chul S Ha Department of Radiation Oncology, University of Texas Health Science Center at San Antonio, and The Cancer Therapy and Research Center, San Antonio, Texas, USA

Mohammad Khan Department of Radiation Oncology, Cleveland Clinic, Cleveland, Ohio, USA

Roger M Macklis Department of Radiation Oncology and Taussig Cancer Center, Cleveland Clinic Lerner College of Medicine, Cleveland, Ohio, USA

Erin S Murphy Department of Radiation Oncology, Cleveland Clinic, Cleveland, Ohio, USA

Nidhi Sharma Department of Diagnostic Radiology, Cleveland Clinic, Cleveland, Ohio, USA

Kevin Stephans Department of Radiation Oncology, Cleveland Clinic, Cleveland, Ohio, USA

John W Sweetenham Taussig Cancer Institute, Cleveland Clinic, Cleveland, Ohio, USA

Stephanie Terezakis Department of Radiation Oncology and Molecular Radiation Sciences, The Sidney Kimmel Comprehensive Cancer Center at Johns Hopkins, Baltimore, Maryland, USA

Joachim Yahalom Department of Radiation Oncology, Memorial Sloan-Kettering Cancer Center, New York, New York, USA

Acknowledgement

Dr Macklis would like to thank the staff and patients in the Department of Radiation Oncology in the Cleveland Clinic Lerner College of Medicine for helpful discussions and resident chart rounds review sessions.

1   Functional Imaging in Image-Guided Radiation Therapy Treatment Planning: The Next Big Step in Lymphoma Radiotherapy

Nidhi Sharma and Roger M Macklis

The development and widespread application of functional imaging studies such as 18F-fluorodeoxyglucose-positron emission tomography (^{18}F-FDG-PET) and PET/computed tomography (CT) are revolutionizing the planning process for radiation medicine. The ability to define metabolic hot spots and zones of increased cellular activity within the overall tumor targets brings new dimensions of clinical information to the more routine data taken from anatomic 3-D imaging studies, such as CT and magnetic resonance imaging (MRI). In addition to the standard structural and anatomic information provided by the 3-D data sets used to illustrate radiologic scans, functional physiologic correlates maybe useful in deciding on dose intensification or de-intensification for individual zones within apparently homogeneous target volumes. The development in the last decade of efficient and widely available platforms for intensity-modulated radiotherapy (IMRT) now allows us to consider hypothetical "dose painting" approaches in which parameters of functional activity, such as the standardized uptake value (SUV), observed at any particular tissue site can be matched to the dosimetric thresholds and control levels possible using inhomogeneous "pencil beam" intensity-modulated radiation beam delivery. The combination of IMRT dose delivery technology and the newer molecular imaging capabilities allow the possibility of near real-time information feedback loops in which a "plan of the week" or even "plan of the day" are chosen based on metabolic patterns observed at that particular time. In essence, this places the concept of biologically guided radiation therapy (RT) within the larger technical realm of adaptive radiotherapy (AR).

The concept and terms involved in "image guidance" and "image-guided radiation therapy" (IGRT) are used in various ways by various authors. In general, IGRT implies that radiation beam trajectories and intensities are selected and adjusted using updated treatment positional targeting information. In this context, IGRT capabilities may be considered a form of AR in which the targeting variables are modified on a time scale appropriate to the change in dimension for the contours of the target or normal tissue. The term "adaptive radiotherapy" is chosen to emphasize the concept that optimal radiotherapy treatment plans may change over time, thereby requiring readjustment of tumor position and external contours change under treatment. For anatomic image modalities, the concept of AR implies that treatment coordinates obtained and optimized on any particular day (i.e., Day 1 of treatment) may be grossly sub-optimal by Day 10 or 30 or 100. The simplest form of AR assumes that the target conformation and external dimensions do not change substantially from day to day even though the overall position of the target isocenter may be relocated in space. In essence, this simplification assumes that the size and shape of the target are unchanging, although the center of mass may change over time requiring the field to be adjusted. This adjustment is called the "offset" measurement and this offset is typically displayed as a set of coordinates representing the x, y and z positional displacements necessary in order to re-optimize the isocenter position. More complex sets of offset coordinates may include partial rotations (pitch and yaw) and other types of fine-tuning related to the dosimetric influences of surrounding structures. At an even higher level of optimization complexity, one can begin to consider change in target morphology, as one might imagine if target segments were growing or shrinking during the course of treatment. For instance, some recent data suggest that the contour of many adenocarcinoma targets may decrease by approximately 1% per day while under radiotherapy. This amount of target shrinkage, though small on a day by day basis, amounts to a significant shrinkage in tissue mass over the course of an entire 7-week period of radiotherapy. This may result in significant decreases in the beam attenuation profile of the target under radiotherapy. For any of these types of changes in positional target registration compared to the baseline location, the possible need to re-plan the case is obvious. Minor registrational offsets may be appropriately corrected using simple isocenter shifts, but more complex perturbations in tissue location may result in dramatic dosimetric differences for both target and nearby normal tissues. This kind of change may thus require complete re-planning of the case and the re-positioning of critical normal structures behind blocks. In some cases, a specific template may be used to develop a family of plans during the initial treatment planning episode. Changes in positional coordinates may then be accommodated by choosing the plan within the treatment library that best accommodates the positional information detected by the day's imaging studies.

The incorporation of functional imaging into the AR paradigm presents another step in the evolution away from utilizing static Day 1 treatment coordinates and beam intensities and towards optimized treatment coordinates and beam intensities defined for later time frames. The use of the serial functional imaging studies and correlated target parameters allows the inclusion of non-positional information to be included within this sort of optimization beam delivery matrix.

Positron Emission Tomography/Computed Tomography Information as a New Critical Treatment Planning Element

Though functional imaging using molecular tracers such as ^{18}F-FDG has been available since the 1960s, this technology has only recently been considered central enough for widespread tumor evaluation. The principles behind ^{18}F-FDG-PET involve changes in glucose metabolism and localization, and abnormalities in glucose metabolism have been known to be characteristic of neoplastic tissue since the 1800s when first investigated by Otto Warburg. This so called "Warburg Effect" was recognized in the 19th century as an unusual pattern of glucose use and sequestration characteristic of many different kinds of cancers. The overall effect appears to relate to three different physiologic perturbations:

1. Increased hexokinase activity observed within tumor cells
2. Increased neoplastic rate of hexose monophosphate shunt activity
3. Changes in glucose transport characteristics on the part of the tumor cell membranes

When these abnormal patterns of tumor physiology are identified, the patterns of glucose localization and trapping within tumor cells often serves as an excellent though non-specific marker of malignancy. The use of ^{18}F-FDG as a glucose analog allows non-invasive monitoring of changes in glucose concentrations over time. For malignant lymphoma, the use of ^{18}F-FDG-PET and PET/CT have been extensively investigated and thus exceptionally well validated. In fact, for many of the most aggressive grades of malignant lymphoma, the use of PET/CT both for staging and for response assessment has now become an important part of the tumor evaluation process. As a result, the standard management algorithms promulgated by the National Comprehensive Cancer Network (NCCN) and other authoritative bodies all now incorporate the use of functional imaging for lymphoma management.

To understand why the ^{18}F-FDG technology is so well suited to malignant lymphoma, one should understand the common clinical questions involved in the management of this tumor group. Of the nearly 10,000 cases of Hodgkin's lymphoma and 60,000 cases of B-cell non-Hodgkin's lymphoma (NHL) seen in the USA yearly, over half will demonstrate ^{18}F-FDG-avid physiology during the initial staging process. In the case of the most aggressive lymphomas, including Hodgkin's lymphoma, ^{18}F-FDG-PET sensitivity levels on the order of 80–90% are routinely demonstrated with specificity of 90–100%. In comparison, the published sensitivity levels for routine CT evaluations in this same patient group involve levels of 80–90% sensitivity with 40–70% specificity. The ^{18}F-FDG-PET study is therefore more sensitive than CT for this clinical group, although specificity may still be lacking. One of the most frequent unknowns in the staging and re-staging process for this clinical cohort involves the fact that many patients will show grossly enlarged lymph glands that will technically qualify as "adenopathy" when read by experienced radiologist. However, even these grossly enlarged lymph nodes may not harbor neoplastic tissue, since a reactive component often accompanies many kinds of malignant lymphomas. Conversely, regions of minimal disease bulk may not exceed established norms for lymph nodes size, but may still show clear-cut ^{18}F-FDG-PET abnormalities and glucose sequestration consistent with lymphomatous involvement [1].

Although no single count-rate normalization process will differentiate tumor from non-tumor based only on patterns of FDG uptake, recent algorithms developed for the SUV are essentially a count-rate normalizing process designed to allow valid subtraction of background levels of FDG uptake in a way that is reasonably specific and useful in differentiating tumor from non-tumor in most cases. False positives are unfortunately common, and this is especially true for tissues that have been subjected to prior inflammatory stresses, including surgery, hyperthermia, ionizing radiation or cytotoxic chemotherapy. Any source of inflammation can cause major increases in SUV levels. Though many clinical studies quote a SUV level of approximately 2.5–3 as the boundary between normal and neoplastic tissue, the use of any single value as a differentiator between cancer and non-cancer is likely to

yield unsatisfactory results. Patient preparation and machine settings may differ dramatically between institutions. The limited sensitivity and specificity of the PET procedure makes it perilous to use any one particular SUV as the sole indicator of malignant potential. For low-grade lymphoma, there is a trend toward lower SUV number, although this pattern is not at all absolute. Hodgkin's lymphoma represents a particularly well studied example and the current guidelines suggest the use of PET both in initial characterization and work up and during subsequent course of care. Many lymphoma investigators insist on a pre-chemotherapy study in order to have a basis line, since patients may differ substantially in their response based on observed ^{18}F-FDG SUV level. A PET/CT study that goes from convincingly positive to convincingly negative is somewhat reassuring with respect to the likelihood of response to treatment. However, studies show that a "negativizing" PET scan cannot be considered a demonstration of tumor cell elimination. In the same way, a patient who has gone from a convincingly positive PET study to a convincingly negative PET study and then shows a recurrence of the high SUV level later in the course of care is certainly a likely suspect for clinical recurrence site.

In addition to the increase in SUV levels caused by post-inflammatory states, certain body tissues also show a spurious increase in SUV. For instance, "brown fat" can appear to be a classic cancer-related FDG hotspot on PET even though there may be no evidence of cancer within the evaluated tissue. The use of PET/CT correlated with high quality diagnostic CT studies is obligatory if one wishes to separate normal from neoplastic tissues under these circumstances (Fig. 1.1).

The use of correlated ^{18}F-FDG-PET/CT studies has contributed significantly to the utility of functional imaging for radiotherapy planning. By allowing fairly precise correlation between the

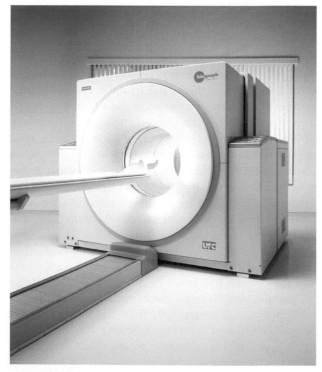

Figure 1.1 A combined positron emission tomography and low dose CT (PET-CT scanner) with uniform high resolution and good image quality.

anatomic location of a particular FDG hotspot and the underlying 3D anatomy as determined by high resolution CT, many equivocal findings can be supported or refuted. Moreover, since most radio-therapy treatment plans rely on the initial planning CT data set to indicate the primary target localizer information, the addition of correlated PET/CT information to the sort of original PET evaluation produced in the 1990s has contributed greatly to the utility of the technology in radiation oncology. Just as MRI data sets are usually incorporated into radiotherapy planning by fusion with the more geometrically precise CT data, the use of corre-lated PET/CT for radiotherapy planning minimizes ambiguities and incorrect evaluations. PET studies have notoriously poor resolution (approximately 0.5 cm at best), thus the registration of the PET information to the much more geometrically accurate CT data set is obligatory. As PET/CT data continues to accumu-late, some have argued we should investigate the concept "dose painting" based on a matrix constructed using the corrected SUV map. Such dose painting would theoretically allow one to iden-tify biologically relevant sub-volumes within the tumor or target tissue contours. These sub-volumes could be planned for dose escalation or diminution compared to baseline doses. Although the concept has great intuitive appeal, the underlying hypoth-esis (i.e., that high SUV levels correspond to "more dangerous" portions of target and therefore need higher radiation doses) has not been well validated. Indeed, areas of relative tumor hypoxia, which should theoretically require higher radiation doses due to the well-described radiobiologic oxygen sensitization effect, would ultimately be detected on ^{18}F-FDG PET studies as cold spots rather than hot spots. The naive use of SUV matrix informa-tion in order to determine individual sub-volumes for radiation dose delivery is therefore exceedingly risky. Should "hot spots" on FDG-PET receive higher or lower doses of radiation? One can design an argument in favor of either course of action. Extensive validation will therefore be necessary.

Another important factor relates to the potentially transient nature of the hypoxic patterns observed. Recent investigations employing the hypoxic cell detector 18F-misonidazole have shown beautiful pictures that appear to correlate with regions of hypoxia. However, these hypoxia patterns are often unstable and therefore may be of minimal use in the selection of an optimized treatment plan. Much additional work will need to be done before radiation dose painting based on ^{18}F-FDG localization becomes reality. The working concept of intensifying dose delivery based on residual post-chemotherapy target cells is, however, innately appealing.

Overall, one can say that the incorporation of functional imaging into modern radiotherapy treatment planning is still a work in progress. Many recent studies have suggested significant changes in planned radiotherapy fields once PET or PET/CT information is included in the imaging data set. Some studies sug-gest that up to 50% of treatment plans will undergo modification once the FDG information is incorporated. However, the plan changes may be such that the net treated volume either increases or decreases. Thus, it is impossible to identify a consistent pattern. The inherent subjectivity of the ^{18}F-FDG-PET study interpretation implies that we are still in the learning phase with respect to how best to incorporate functional imaging data into dose delivery strategies. Although IGRT clearly provides a mechanism for inho-mogeneous dose delivery, the decision on whether to either inten-sify or de-intensify dose at any particular sub-volume based on a single set of ^{18}F-FDG-PET images must be clarified and validated prior to clinical implementation. The individualized treatment of malignant lymphoma will probably be a prime proving ground for the underlying hypotheses behind selective target sub-contouring and dose delivery based on functional imaging studies.

REFERENCE

1. PET/CT in Radiation Oncology: The FROG Manual for clinical use. 2nd edn.

2 Role of ^{18}F-fluorodeoxyglucose Positron Emission Tomography/Computed Tomography in the Evaluation and Management of Lymphoma

Dominique Delbeke, Angelika Bischof Delaloye and Peter S Conti

Introduction

^{18}F-fluorodeoxyglucose (^{18}F-FDG) positron emission tomography/computed tomography (PET/CT) is an imaging modality combining anatomical imaging with CT and metabolic imaging with PET, using ^{18}F-FDG as a radiopharmaceutical. ^{18}F-FDG PET/CT has become an established modality for evaluation of patients with malignancies, including patients with lymphoma.

Recommendations for the clinical use of ^{18}F-FDG PET/CT imaging are now available [1] and ^{18}F-FDG PET/CT imaging has been incorporated in the management algorithms recommended by the National Comprehensive Cancer Network (NCCN) [2]. Procedures and practice guidelines have been published by both the Society of Nuclear Medicine (SNM) and the American College of Radiology (ACR) [3–4]. Recommendations regarding the use of ^{18}F-FDG PET in National Cancer Institute (NCI) clinical trials are also available [5]. For patients with lymphoma, consensus recommendations regarding the use of ^{18}F-FDG PET for assessment response has been published by the imaging subcommittee of the International Harmonization Project (IHP), including criteria for interpretation [6]. Response criteria for lymphoma have been revised based on PET/CT imaging, eliminating the "complete remission unconfirmed (CRu)" category [7].

This segment of the book will review: (1) some basic concepts of ^{18}F-FDG and PET/CT imaging; (2) the literature supporting the use of ^{18}F-FDG PET and PET/CT in the evaluation of patients with lymphoma; and (3) the guidelines and recommendations for the use of ^{18}F-FDG PET and PET/CT in the evaluation of patients with lymphoma.

Basic Concepts of ^{18}F-FDG and PET/CT Imaging

Physiological Variations of ^{18}F-FDG Distribution

^{18}F-FDG is an analog of glucose and behaves as a tracer of glucose metabolism. Therefore, the distribution of ^{18}F-FDG is not limited to malignant tissue. ^{18}F-FDG enters into cells by the same transport mechanism as glucose and is then intracellularly phosphorylated by a hexokinase into ^{18}F-FDG-6-phosphate (^{18}F-FDG-6-P). In tissues with a low concentration of glucose-6-phosphatase, such as the brain, the myocardium and most malignant cells, ^{18}F-FDG-6-P does not enter into further enzymatic pathways, but accumulates intracellularly proportional to the glycolytic rate. Some tissues, such as the liver, kidney, intestine, muscle and some malignant cells, have varying degrees of glucose-6-phosphatase activity, and do not accumulate ^{18}F-FDG-6-P to the same extent.

To interpret ^{18}F-FDG images, the interpreter must be familiar with the normal distribution of ^{18}F-FDG, physiological variations and benign conditions associated with ^{18}F-FDG accumulation [8,9].

The cortex of the brain uses glucose as its only substrate, therefore, ^{18}F-FDG accumulation is normally high. The myocardium, on the other hand, can use various substrates according to substrate availability and hormonal status. In the fasting state, the myocardium utilizes free fatty acids, but after a glucose load it favors glucose. When the thorax is evaluated with ^{18}F-FDG to assess the presence of malignant lesions, a 12-hour fast is recommended to avoid artifacts due to myocardial activity. For evaluation of coronary artery disease, a glucose load with or without insulin supplementation is usually given to promote myocardial uptake of ^{18}F-FDG. Unlike glucose, ^{18}F-FDG is excreted by the kidneys, and focal ureteral accumulation should not be mistaken for a malignant lesion. Concentration of ^{18}F-FDG in the renal collecting system may obscure the evaluation of that region. This can be minimized by maintaining good hydration and by the administration of loop diuretics. For adequate visualization of the pelvis, irrigation of the bladder via a urinary catheter can be useful.

At rest, skeletal muscle uptake of ^{18}F-FDG is low, but after exercise, a significant accumulation of ^{18}F-FDG in selected muscle groups may be misleading. For example, in the evaluation of the head and neck, uptake in the muscles of mastication or laryngeal muscles may mimic malignant lesions. Therefore, it is important for the patient to avoid strenuous exercise 24 hours prior to ^{18}F-FDG administration and during the uptake phase following ^{18}F-FDG injection, including chewing or talking. Hyperventilation may induce uptake in the diaphragm, and anxiety-induced muscle uptake is often seen in the trapezius and paraspinal muscles. Muscle relaxants, such as benzodiazepines, may be helpful in anxious patients. ^{18}F-FDG uptake can also occur in metabolically active adipose tissue (brown fat), particularly in young individuals and cold environment. The distribution is usually typical and includes bilateral neck, supraclavicular regions, anterior mediastinum, axillae, paravertebral regions and suprarenal fossae. Temperature control or the administration of beta-blockers reduce brown adipose tissue uptake.

Another source of misinterpretation is uptake in the gastrointestinal tract. There is usually uptake in the lymphoid tissue of Waldeyer's ring, and prominent uptake in the cecum of many patients may also be related to abundant lymphoid tissue in the intestinal wall. Uptake in smooth muscle can also be seen with active peristalsis and ^{18}F-FDG is secreted in the lumen of the intestine. The wall of the stomach is often faintly seen and can be used as an anatomical landmark; similarly, activity is frequently seen at the gastro-esophageal junction. More prominent ^{18}F-FDG uptake is seen when inflammatory changes are present, such as in esophagitis, gastritis and inflammatory bowel disease.

Physiologic thymic uptake may be present in children and in patients after chemotherapy. Its typical smooth, symmetrical V-shape usually allows differentiation from residual lymphoma.

Marked diffuse bone marrow and splenic uptake is often seen after chemotherapy, especially if colony-stimulating factors are administered concurrently, and may compromise evaluation of the marrow for malignant involvement. This is due to bone marrow hyperplasia and extramedullary hematopoiesis. Marrow uptake returns to normal 4–6 weeks after completion of chemotherapy.

^{18}F-FDG is taken up by activated macrophages at sites of inflammation, and the uptake may often be sufficient to resemble malignant lesions when there is granulomatous inflammation, such as with tuberculosis, sarcoidosis, fungal infections and aspergillosis.

In order to avoid misinterpretation of ^{18}F-FDG images, it is critical to standardize the environment of the patient during the uptake period, to examine the patient for post-operative site, drainage tubes, stoma, etc., and to time ^{18}F-FDG imaging appropriately after invasive procedures and therapies. Although ^{18}F-FDG shares some of the limitations of other tumor imaging agents, such as ^{67}Ga, ^{201}Tl and ^{99m}Tc-MIBI, the relatively high ratio of tumor-to-non-tumor activity observed in most malignant lesions accounts for the reported high sensitivity and specificity of ^{18}F-FDG imaging and the intrinsic characteristics of PET imaging.

Integrated ^{18}F-FDG PET/CT Imaging

A summary of literature regarding the performance of ^{18}F-FDG PET in various malignancies was published in 2001 [10].

Although numerous studies have shown that the sensitivity and specificity of ^{18}F-FDG imaging may be superior to that of CT in many clinical settings, the inability of ^{18}F-FDG imaging to provide anatomical localization remained a significant impairment in maximizing its clinical utility. Additional limitations of ^{18}F-FDG PET imaging include the limited resolution of PET systems compared to CT and physiological variations of ^{18}F-FDG distribution.

Limitations of anatomical imaging with CT are well-known and related to size criteria to differentiate benign from malignant lymph nodes, difficulty differentiating post-therapy changes from tumor recurrence and difficulty differentiating non-opacified loops of bowel from malignant lesions in the abdomen and pelvis.

Close correlation of ^{18}F-FDG studies with conventional CT scans helps to minimize these difficulties and interpretation has traditionally been accomplished by visually comparing corresponding ^{18}F-FDG and CT images. To aid in image interpretation, computer software has been developed to co-register the ^{18}F-FDG PET emission images with the high-resolution anatomical images provided by CT.

An alternative approach that has gained wider acceptance is the introduction of multimodality imaging with integrated PET/CT. Design innovations continue to be developed.

Integrated PET/CT Systems

The fusion of anatomical and molecular images (PET and CT) obtained with integrated PET/CT systems, sequentially in time but without moving the patient from the imaging table, allows optimal co-registration of anatomic and molecular images leading to accurate attenuation correction and precise anatomic localization of lesions with increased metabolism. The fusion images provided by these systems allow the most accurate interpretation of both PET/CT studies in oncology. Fusion ^{18}F-FDG PET/CT imaging is also a promising tool for optimizing radiation therapy.

Published data regarding the incremental value of integrated PET/CT compared to PET alone, or PET correlated with a CT obtained at a different time conclude the following: (1) improvement of lesion detection on both CT and PET images; (2) improvement of the localization of foci of uptake, resulting in better differentiation physiologic from pathologic uptake; and (3) precise localization of the malignant foci, e.g., in the skeleton versus soft tissue, or liver versus adjacent bowel or node.

PET/CT fusion images affect clinical management by (1) guiding further procedures, (2) excluding the need for further procedures, and (3) changing both inter- and intra-modality therapy. PET/CT fusion images have the potential to provide important information to guide the biopsy of a mass to active regions of the tumor and to provide better maps than CT alone to modulate field and dose of radiation therapy.[11]

Technical issues regarding optimal protocols and technical and clinical expertise regarding performance and interpretation of PET/CT imaging have been discussed [3]. Procedure guidelines for tumor imaging using ^{18}F-FDG PET/CT have also been published and list numerous sources of false-positive and false-negative findings [4]. This new powerful technology provides more accurate interpretation of both CT and PET images and, therefore, more optimal patient care.

Visual versus Semi-Quantitative Interpretation of ^{18}F-FDG PET/CT Images

Evaluation of PET images can be performed visually or semi-quantitatively using the standard uptake value (SUV) or the ratio of uptake between a lesion and an internal reference organ, such as blood pool or normal hepatic parenchyma (average SUV ~2.0). Although semi-quantitative assessment offers a more objective estimation of the metabolic activity of the lesions, visual analysis may be adequate for clinical purposes in most instances.

The SUV is the activity in the lesion in microCi/ml (kBq/ml) corrected for the weight of the patient and the activity of ^{18}F-FDG administered. The SUV may be more accurate when measured relative to body surface area or lean body mass than body weight. The average SUV of normal liver parenchyma and blood pool is approximately 2.0 and can be used as a visual reference.

The SUV depends on accurate calibration of the PET system, accurate soft tissue attenuation correction, and reconstruction algorithms among other factors.

Accurate SUV determination also depends on accurate attenuation correction. As CT-transmission maps are acquired just before the acquisition of the emission data, attenuation correction can be compromised by imperfect registration of the transmission and emission scans due to patient motion.

The SUV is also dependent on factors that are difficult to control in the clinical environment, such as the patient's plasma glucose and insulin levels, fasting state, dose infiltration, recent physical activity and uptake time of ^{18}F-FDG. In addition, there is inter- and intra-observer variability in identification of the lesion and slice with highest uptake and in drawing contours around the regions of interest. Therefore, comparison of SUVs between two studies in the same patient for assessing response to therapy requires rigorous quality control, especially if performed on different PET systems, or using different protocols and variation between institutions.

General Indications for ^{18}F-FDG PET/CT Imaging

It is well established that neoplastic cells demonstrate increased metabolic activity. This is due, in part, to an increased density of glucose transporter proteins and increased intracellular glycolytic enzyme levels. Although variations in uptake are known to exist among tumor types, elevated uptake of ^{18}F-FDG has been demonstrated in most malignant primary tumors including lymphomas. Therefore, the most common indications for ^{18}F-FDG imaging are:

1. Differentiation of benign from malignant lesions
2. Staging and restaging malignant lesions
3. Detection of malignant recurrence
4. Monitoring response to therapy

^{18}F-FDG PET and PET/CT in the Evaluation of Lymphoma

Degree of ^{18}F-FDG Avidity of Different Types of Lymphoma

Lymphomas are classified into two main groups, non-Hodgkin's lymphomas (NHL) and Hodgkin's lymphoma (HL). NHL is more common than HL, representing approximately 85% of lymphomas.

Hodgkin's Lymphoma. The World Health Organization (WHO) classifies HL as classical with four classical subtypes (nodular sclerosis, mixed cellularity, lymphocyte rich, lymphocyte-depleted) and as nodular lymphocyte-predominant HL (NLPHL), the latter representing about 5% of all cases. HL is virtually always intensively ^{18}F-FDG avid [12]. NLPHL with a mean SUV maximum of 9.3 ($n=7$) has the best prognosis, nodular sclerosing (NS) HL is the most common subtype with a mean SUV maximum of 16.3 ($n=36$), mixed cellularity HL (MCHL) has a worse prognosis than NS with a SUV maximum of 20.8 ($n=11$), and lymphocyte-depleted HL has the worst prognosis.

Non-Hodgkin's Lymphoma. According to the WHO [13,14], NHL are classified histologically into more than 30 subtypes of (1) B-cell neoplasms and (2) T-cell/natural killer (NK)-cell neoplasms.

The NHLs can also be divided into two prognostic groups: the indolent lymphomas and the aggressive lymphomas [15]. Indolent NHL types have a relatively good prognosis, with median survival as long as 10 years, but they are usually not curable in advanced clinical stages. Follicular lymphoma (FL) is the most common type of indolent lymphoma, representing 22% of NHL. Marginal zone B-cell lymphoma and chronic lymphocytic leukemia/small lymphocytic lymphoma (CLL/SLL) are other types of indolent lymphoma each representing 6–8% of NHL. Diffuse large B-cell lymphoma (DLBCL) is the most common aggressive lymphoma representing 30% of NHL; other relatively common aggressive lymphomas include mantle cell lymphoma (MCL) and adult T-cell leukemia/lymphoma, each representing 6–8% of NHL.

Although there is an overlap of SUV between aggressive and indolent NHL, on average the SUVs in aggressive NHL and HL are higher than those obtained for indolent lymphomas [16]. In a study of 97 patients with NHL untreated for 6 months, indolent lymphomas had a SUV of 7.0±3.1 (mean±SD) compared to a SUV of 19.6±9.3 (mean±SD) for aggressive lymphomas. Despite the overlap, all indolent lymphomas had a SUV smaller than 13 and all aggressive lymphomas had a SUV greater than 13. A SUV greater than 10 excluded indolent lymphoma with a specificity of 81%.

Two studies of 172 and 255 patients, respectively, have evaluated the sensitivity of ^{18}F-FDG PET for detection of HL and NHL according to histology: most aggressive NHL was intensively ^{18}F-FDG avid [17,18]. The sensitivity ranges were as follows: HL, DLBCL and MCL: 98–100%, FL: 91–98%, marginal zone lymphoma: 67–82%, peripheral T-cell lymphoma: 40% and CLL/SLL: 50%.

Other studies have reported a more variable degree of ^{18}F-FDG avidity in MCL [19] and T-cell lymphoma [20]. ^{18}F-FDG PET is usually positive with higher SUVs seen in NK T-cell lymphomas compared to peripheral T-cell lymphomas.

SLL/CLL and extranodal marginal zone B-cell lymphoma are low-grade lymphomas and are often poorly ^{18}F-FDG avid, unless they undergo transformation to a more aggressive subtype (Richter transformation) [21,22]. In a study comparing conventional modalities and ^{18}F-FDG PET, the sensitivity of ^{18}F-FDG PET was 58% for detection of SLL/CLL. In patients with Richter transformation into DLBCL, the sensitivity was 91%. In addition, ^{18}F-FDG PET can guide biopsy to the sites of high-grade transformation.

The sensitivity of FDG PET is reportedly higher in nodal marginal zone lymphoma compared to extranodal marginal B-cell lymphoma, probably due to the differences in disease behavior between these two entities [23,24].

^{18}F-FDG PET and PET/CT for Diagnosing Lymphoma

In patients presenting with lymphadenopathy or mediastinal masses, the differential diagnosis includes lymphoma or other malignancies, and inflammatory/infectious etiologies. Both malignant and inflammatory etiologies (especially granulomatous) can be ^{18}F-FDG avid, as ^{18}F-FDG is a marker of glucose metabolism.

However, in patients with suspected lymphoma, ^{18}F-FDG PET may be indicated in certain clinical settings and helpful in finding the most appropriate site for biopsy. In patients with lymphoma, ^{18}F-FDG uptake can be heterogenous in the same patient, presumably representing different clones of cells with different glucose metabolism and different biologic behavior. ^{18}F-FDG PET can guide biopsy to the site of maximum ^{18}F-FDG uptake, representing the most aggressive portion of the tumor.

^{18}F-FDG PET is also useful in the evaluation of primary central nervous system (CNS) lymphoma. This is particularly true for human immunodeficiency virus (HIV)-positive patients who are at greater risk for occurrence of CNS lymphoma than the general population. Primary lymphoma of the CNS is rare, representing 1–3% of all primary brain tumors. Most are DLBCL, which are intensely ^{18}F-FDG avid and may be appreciated even against the generally high physiological uptake of normal cerebral tissue. Common sites of occurrence are the cerebral hemispheres, basal ganglia and corpus callosum [25].

HIV-positive patients are also at an increased risk for opportunistic infections, including toxoplasmosis of the brain. CNS lymphoma and cerebral toxoplasmosis can be indistinguishable on CT or magnetic resonance imaging (MRI) imaging. Accurate and rapid distinction between these two entities is paramount, since prompt and appropriate treatment for either of these diagnoses is essential for a favorable outcome. Unlike CT or MRI, ^{18}F-FDG PET/CT can usually distinguish between CNS lymphoma and toxoplasmosis infection, with CNS lymphoma typically being intensely ^{18}F-FDG avid, relative to normal cerebral uptake, whereas infection from toxoplasmosis is usually not. ^{18}F-FDG PET can differentiate lymphomas of the CNS from infectious processes with an accuracy of 89% [26–27]. In addition, using ^{18}F-FDG PET/CT to target the biopsy to the site of maximum activity increases the biopsy accuracy by decreasing biopsy sampling error.

Whole body ^{18}F-FDG PET/CT is also useful in the initial staging of CNS lymphoma with occult sites of systemic disease found in up to 15% of patients who are otherwise believed to have disease confined to the CNS [28]. Restaging can also be performed with ^{18}F-FDG PET/CT to evaluate for persistent or recurrent metabolically active disease.

^{18}F-FDG PET and PET/CT for Staging of Lymphoma
Ann Arbor Staging. Ann Arbor staging is the universally accepted staging system for lymphomas [14]. This system is based on the distribution and number of involved sites, as well as the presence or absence of extranodal involvement and constitutional symptoms. Stages I–IV adult lymphomas can be subclassified into A and B categories: B for those with defined general symptoms and A for those without B symptoms. The designation E is used when there is localized extranodal lymphoma near the major lymphatic aggregates. Lymphomas originate from extralymphatic organs in up to 30% of patients.

Stage I and II (lymph node involvement only on one side of the diaphragm) have a high cure rate, whereas stage III (lymph node involvement on both sides of the diaphragm) and IV (systemic involvement) have a lower cure rate.

For NHL and HL, the frequency of involvement of the spleen is ~22%, liver is 15 and 3%, respectively, and bone marrow is 25 and 10%, respectively.

Prognostic Value of ^{18}F-FDG PET. High degree of ^{18}F-FDG uptake pre-therapy indicates a worse prognosis. In a study of 34 patients with untreated lymphoma and a follow-up 15–50 months after starting therapy, patients with recurrence had higher SUV pre-therapy than patients in remission. The SUV was 6.4 ± 3.0 (mean$\pm$SD) in patients in complete remission and no recurrence, the SUV was 7.0 ± 2.9 (mean$\pm$SD) in patients who went into complete remission, then recurred, and the SUV was 14.4 ± 5.5 (mean$\pm$SD) in patients with no remission. Survival was longer for patients with SUV smaller than 8.0 [29].

^{18}F-FDG PET for Staging Lymphoma: Comparison with [67]Ga Scintigraphy. In comparison to ^{67}Ga scintigraphy, ^{18}F-FDG PET has a superior accuracy and is usually positive at the majority of disease sites, while ^{67}Ga single photon emission computed tomography (SPECT) may fail to demonstrate uptake in approximately 25% of disease sites, regardless of the size, disease location and histology in both nodal and extranodal disease [30–31]. The patient sensitivity for ^{18}F-FDG PET and ^{67}Ga scintigraphy is 87–100% and 63–80%, respectively. Therefore, ^{18}F-FDG PET has supplanted ^{67}Ga imaging of patients with lymphoma.

^{18}F-FDG PET and PET/CT for Detection of Nodal and Extranodal Lymphoma. ^{18}F-FDG is the metabolic tracer of choice for imaging of lymphoma. It is highly sensitive and superior to CT in detecting nodal and extranodal involvement in most histologic subtypes of lymphoma [32,33].

A study of 52 patients compared the performance of ^{18}F-FDG PET to CT using the receiver-operator curve (ROC) analysis [34]. The performance of PET was superior to CT for detection of both nodal and extranodal involvement on both sides of the diaphragm. For detection of bone marrow involvement, PET was equivalent to bone marrow biopsy and both were superior to CT. PET changed stage and management in 8% of patients.

In a meta-analysis of 14 of 20 studies selected with 854 patients with lymphoma, the median sensitivity for detection of lymphoma was 90%, the median specificity was 90% and the pooled false-positive rate was 10%. The maximum joint sensitivity and specificity was 88% [35].

Many studies have shown the superiority of PET compared to CT for detection of extranodal involvement because organomegaly is not always associated with disease involvement. ^{18}F-FDG PET has been shown to be more sensitive than CT, identifying 23% more hepatic and splenic lesions [37,36,37].

^{18}F-FDG PET/CT for Detection of Bone Marrow Involvement by Lymphoma. For detection of bone marrow involvement, ^{18}F-FDG PET is more accurate than CT [38,39]. Bone marrow biopsy suffers from sampling error, and ^{18}F-FDG PET can guide the biopsy to ^{18}F-FDG-avid lesions. A prospective evaluation of 78 untreated patients (39 HD, 39 NHL) compared PET and bilateral posterior iliac crest biopsy. PET and biopsy were concordant in 64 patients, biopsy was positive and PET negative in 4 patients, and biopsy was negative and PET positive in 10 patients. A repeat PET-guided biopsy was positive in 8 of these 10 patients. The false-negative PET results were in patients with low-grade lymphomas. PET changed staging in 10% (8/78) of these patients.

A meta-analysis of 13 studies with 587 patients comparing ^{18}F-FDG PET to bone marrow biopsy demonstrated an overall sensitivity of 51% and specificity of 91% [40]. In this study also, 6 of 12 patients with positive ^{18}F-FDG PET and negative bone marrow biopsy, had a positive repeat PET-guided biopsy. Analysis of subgroups of patients demonstrated that ^{18}F-FDG PET was more sensitive for HL and aggressive lymphomas. ^{18}F-FDG PET is complimentary but cannot replace bone marrow biopsy because of the false-negative rate, especially in low-grade lymphoma.

^{18}F-FDG PET criteria for diffuse involvement of the spleen or bone marrow is uptake more intense than in normal liver parenchyma, which has an average SUV of ~2.0 [7].

The diffuse pattern of uptake of reactive bone marrow hyperplasia after chemotherapy, and especially after concurrent administration of bone marrow stimulants, can mimic or mask diffuse bone marrow involvement. Therefore, appropriate history is critical. A delay of 3–4 weeks after completion of therapy permits the physiologic marrow activity to abate [7].

^{18}F-FDG PET versus ^{18}F-FDG PET/CT and CT Protocol for ^{18}F-FDG PET/CT. PET/CT is commonly performed without intravenous contrast and a low-dose (40–80 mAs) CT component to reduce the radiation dose to the patient. When the protocol for the CT component is not specified, the low-dose CT without intravenous contrast is usually applied. However, the CT component can be performed using a diagnostic CT protocol with oral and intravenous contrast.

A study of 27 patients with lymphoma, using 12 months follow-up as standard of reference, demonstrated that the sensitivity of ^{18}F-FDG PET/CT with fusion images for detection of lymphoma was superior to PET and CT side by side, PET alone and CT alone on patient- and lesion-based analysis. The sensitivity of PET/CT was 93% (patient) and 96% (lesion) compared to 93% (patient) and 91% (lesion) for PET and CT side by side, 86% (patient) and 78% (lesion) for PET alone, and 78% (patient) and 61% (lesion) for CT alone [41]. These conclusions were supported by a similar study [42].

PET/low-dose CT and contrast-enhanced CT (ceCT) performed within 24 days were compared in 60 patients with lymphoma (HL=42, NHL=18) [43]. The sensitivity and specificity of PET/CT was superior to ceCT for detection of lymph node and organ involvement by lymphoma. For lymph node involvement, the sensitivity was 94% and specificity was 100% for PET/CT compared to a sensitivity of 88% and a specificity of 86% for ceCT. For organ involvement, the sensitivity was 88% and specificity was 100% for PET/CT compared to a sensitivity of 50% and specificity of 90% for ceCT. The agreement between PET/CT and ceCT was excellent for detection of lymph node involvement and poor for detection of organ involvement.

PET/low-dose CT and ceCT were compared regarding the change of stage and management in 103 patients referred for initial staging of lymphoma (HL=35, NHL=68) [44]. PET/CT changed the stage in 32% of patients with NHL (31% upstaged, 1% downstaged) and 47% of patients with HL (32% upstaged and 15% downstaged). PET/CT changed the management of 25 and 45% of patients with NHL and HL, respectively.

PET/low-dose CT and PET/ceCT were compared in 47 patients with lymphoma. On a region-based analysis, there was no significant difference for detection of lymphoma. PET/ceCT provided slightly less equivocal sites (2/188) and allowed detection of slightly more extranodal sites (n=4/188). For the purpose of staging, there was almost perfect agreement (46/47 patients) [45].

These three studies concluded that PET/low-dose CT may be adequate for most patients and that ceCT may be recommended for selected cases.

The imaging subcommittee of the IHP recommends the use of ^{18}F-FDG PET in addition to/or integrated with ceCT for initial staging [7]. After therapy, PET should be complemented with CT using a low-dose CT protocol if there was no liver/spleen involvement at baseline and ceCT if there was liver/spleen involvement at baseline.

Impact of ^{18}F-FDG PET/CT on Management of Patients with Lymphoma. The change of stage I/II to III/IV has major therapeutic implications. A change of stage and management has been reported in various studies summarized in a review paper [46]. Although a change in stage due to ^{18}F-FDG PET has been reported in 20–40% of patients, major change of management occurs only in 10–35%, when patients are upstaged from stage I/II to III/IV. Besides staging, pre-treatment PET is indicated to assess FDG avidity of the tumor, especially in lymphoma subtypes with variable FDG uptake patterns.

^{18}F-FDG PET and PET/CT for Monitoring Therapy of Lymphoma
An important indication of PET/CT is monitoring the response to treatment of NHL as well as HL by following the tumor uptake of ^{18}F-FDG [47]. Other radiopharmaceuticals than ^{18}F-FDG might ultimately play a role, but are not yet in routine clinical use and therefore are not part of the present evaluation [48,49].

Differentiation of Viable Tumor from Residual Masses. Since the late 1990s, the value of ^{18}F-FDG PET in differentiating viable tumor from residual masses on CT after first-line treatment is well known [50,51]. Subsequently, it could be shown that adding the results of ^{18}F-FDG PET to currently used International Workshop Criteria (IWC) significantly improved response assessment [52,53]. In particular, ^{18}F-FDG PET was able to identify a significant number of patients considered as having achieved unconfirmed complete (CRu) or partial remission (PR) by IWC criteria, who showed no uptake of ^{18}F-FDG and whose progression-free survival (PFS) was comparable to patients considered in CR. Consequently, it was proposed to revise the response criteria for lymphoma by integrating IWC, mostly based on CT evaluation using RECIST (response evaluation criteria in solid tumors) adapted to lymphoma, and ^{18}F-FDG PET, including immunohistochemistry (IHC) and flow cytometry.[8] According to these revised response criteria (Table 2.1), CR is defined by negative PET of ^{18}F-FDG-avid or pre-treatment PET-positive lymphomas, the absence of palpable spleen and lymph nodes, as well as a cleared bone marrow on repeat biopsy, confirmed by IHC if indeterminate by morphology. DLBCL and HL, as well as FL and MCL are usually ^{18}F-FDG avid, other aggressive and indolent NHL have variable ^{18}F-FDG uptake and need to be scanned before treatment. In case of unknown or absent ^{18}F-FDG uptake on the pre-treatment scan of such patients, all masses have to show complete regression on CT. This definition shows that ^{18}F-FDG PET is the leading criterion for assessing CR in the vast majority of malignant lymphomas.

These response criteria were originally developed as surrogate response markers for clinical trials, but are now more often used for clinical patient management.

Prognostic Impact of ^{18}F-FDG PET. Early assessment of response to treatment has been found to have major prognostic impact [54,55]. Most of the early studies had a retrospective design and were performed with PET and not PET/CT, but concordantly demonstrated high accuracy in predicting outcome, both for HL and NHL. In an overview of studies evaluating response after one or several cycles, an overall sensitivity for predicting treatment failure of 79% with corresponding specificity of 92% (accuracy 85%) and positive and negative predictive values (PPV and NPV) of 90 and 81%, respectively, has been reported. Another systematic review, published recently [56], comes to somewhat less clear-cut conclusions when evaluating the response evaluated by ^{18}F-FDG PET at completion of therapy. They found reported ranges for sensitivity of 50–100% and 33–77% for HL and NHL, respectively, with corresponding specificities of 67–100% and 82–100% for predicting outcome. These authors conclude that ^{18}F-FDG PET seems to have good accuracy for assessing residual disease in HL. Due to methodological weaknesses of current literature, however, accuracy might be overestimated. They suggest that caution should be used in clinical decision making with respect to the lack of robust evidence of the prognostic value of post-therapy ^{18}F-FDG PET results and advocate the necessity of prospective studies.

It seems intriguing that ^{18}F-FDG PET performed after the first one to four courses of chemotherapy has a higher prospective value than end of treatment PET. It has been shown [57] that ^{18}F-FDG PET after one single cycle of chemotherapy predicted outcome in patients with HL and DLBCL. NPV of ^{18}F-FDG

PET after one cycle was higher than at end of treatment evaluation (100 vs. 91.4%), albeit the difference did not reach statistical significance ($p=0.40$). Among the larger series, some differences can be noticed. In a study of 70 patients with aggressive NHL evaluated at mid-treatment by PET, response to treatment was defined as presence or absence of ^{18}F-FDG uptake on non-attenuation corrected PET [58]. None of the 33 patients with residual ^{18}F-FDG uptake experienced durable remission, whereas 31 of the 37 ^{18}F-FDG negative patients had favorable outcome. Two-year PFS was 4 and 85%, respectively. To overcome some difficulties in interpretation of "negativity", the response category of minimal residual uptake (MRU) was introduced [59]. In a series of 121 patients with aggressive NHL, a 5-year PFS of 89, 59 and 16% for patients with no, minimal or positive ^{18}F-FDG PET, respectively, was observed. Subsequent prospective studies have confirmed these results. In a prospective study including 90 patients with aggressive NHL, 2-year PFS was 82% if ^{18}F-FDG uptake had disappeared (54 patients) after two cycles of chemotherapy, whereas in the remaining 36 patients, it was only 43%; 2-year overall survival (OS) was 90 and 61% in these two groups [60]. Both differences were highly significant. Similar results are available for HL. A prospective multicenter trial included 190 patients with advanced-stage disease (stage IIB–IVB) and 70 patients with stage IIA HL with adverse prognostic factors [61]. All but 11 patients were treated with standard ABVD therapy followed by consolidation radiotherapy in case of bulky presentation or residual tumor mass, independently of the results of ^{18}F-FDG PET performed after two courses of ABVD. Two-year PFS was 13 and 95% for patients with positive and negative interim PET, respectively. In univariate analysis, outcome was significantly associated with interim PET, stage IV disease, WBC >15,000, lymphopenia, international prognostic score (IPS), extranodal involvement and bulky disease. In multivariate analyses, only the results of PET remained significant. The authors conclude that interim ^{18}F-FDG PET is the single most important tool for planning risk-adapted treatment in advanced HL. Another prospective study in 77 consecutive patients with newly diagnosed HL found that interim ^{18}F-FDG PET at two cycles was as accurate as later during treatment and stronger than established prognostic factors [62].

Cell Response after Chemotherapy. The disappearance of ^{18}F-FDG uptake after the first course of chemotherapy indicates chemosensitivity of the tumor, thus predicting outcome. It is, however, not synonymous with the absence of viable tumor cells and therefore does not exclude residual disease. In MCF-7 breast cancer cells submitted to cytotoxic treatment (doxorubicin, 5-FU). in vitro decline of ^{3}H-FDG uptake, after 24 hours, exceeded the decrease of viable tumor cells despite the rise of GLUT-1 mRNA levels. The decrease of hexokinase II mRNA seemed to have a more direct impact on ^{3}H-FDG uptake. Two to four days after treatment, this initial stunning effect disappeared and a strong relationship between ^{3}H-FDG uptake and viable cell number remained, thus supporting the use of ^{18}F-FDG to monitor cancer treatment [63].

Most chemotherapy regimens produce only one log tumor mass reduction per cycle (90%), effective treatment may require up to 10 cycles of chemotherapy. Two cycles of chemotherapy, on average, reduce the cell number to 10^8–10^9 cells corresponding to 0.3–1 cm diameter nodes and therefore to the limit of detection of lymphoma containing nodes with PET. Accordingly, lesions with persistent uptake of ^{18}F-FDG after two cycles of chemotherapy are unlikely to be cured by six additional cycles of chemotherapy, whereas lesions that no longer show uptake may be cured during subsequent chemotherapy. This partially explains the superiority of early ^{18}F-FDG PET versus end-treatment evaluation for assessment of outcome [64].

Pitfalls in Interpretation of ^{18}F-FDG PET/CT in Patients with Lymphoma
False-positive results may hamper the role of early PET. There are physiological and pathological as well as technical and methodological reasons for false-positive studies. The presence of mass lesions by itself may contribute to some visible ^{18}F-FDG uptake on PET. SUV combined with some tumor volume adjustment might refine the interpretation [65]. Besides the well-known reasons for ^{18}F-FDG uptake in non-tumor tissue, such as brown adipose tissue, inflammatory lesions, granulomatous disease, particularly sarcoidosis, thymus, fractures, normal bowel and urinary tract, degenerative joints, normal bone marrow, muscles, contaminations, etc. that are most often easily recognized, especially with PET/CT [66], particular situations can occur in patients treated for lymphoma.

Physiological uptake in response to therapy can occasionally confuse interpretation. Reactive diffuse bone marrow hyperplasia and splenic uptake occur typically for 2–4 weeks after chemotherapy and can be intense after administration of marrow-stimulating factors such as filgrastim [67,68].

Thymic hyperplasia is common in children and young adults with an incidence of 16% [69]. It typically occurs 2–6 months after completion of therapy and may persist for 12–24 months. The pattern of moderate ^{18}F-FDG uptake and the inverted V-shape are typical for thymic hyperplasia.

Under chemotherapy, patients may quite frequently develop pulmonary infiltrates of an inflammatory, toxic or infectious nature, which is not usually suspicious for lymphoma, except in case of pulmonary involvement at diagnosis.

Aggressive NHL is currently most treated by immunochemotherapy such as rituximob. Part of the anti-tumor efficacy of the anti-CD20 antibody may be due to the prolonged recruitment of inflammatory cells in the tumor. This could contribute to persistent ^{18}F-FDG uptake in residual masses and nodes. In an ongoing vaccination trial in patients with FL using dendritic cells loaded with tumor antigens ex vivo [70], a marked increase of ^{18}F-FDG uptake was initially observed in malignant lymph nodes that subsequently disappeared in a patient who ultimately achieved CR. This finding suggests that ^{18}F-FDG may detect induced cell activation and migration of immune cells to tumor [71]. In patients treated with radioimmunotherapy, due to the prolonged action of this type of therapy, response evaluation is usually performed not earlier than 3 months after administration of the radiolabeled antibody [72,73].

Criteria for Interpretation of Response to Therapy
The lack of clearly defined interpretation criteria adds to the difficulty of appraisal. Truly quantitative measures are not conceivable for routine assessment of ^{18}F-FDG uptake. Therefore, most centers

rely on semi-quantitative SUV measurements. Most of the time, comparisons within the same center and for the same patient used as their own control can be quite reliably performed as long as the interval between injection and acquisition and blood glucose levels are comparable, that there is no extravasation during injection of the radiopharmaceutical and the quality control of the instruments (PET, CT, dose calibrator) is regularly performed with consistent results. It is much more delicate to compare SUV obtained in different centers, with different instruments. Therefore, qualitative visual interpretation is most often used in evaluating response for this patient group.

The IHP has published recommendations for appropriate interpretation of response to treatment in patients with lymphoma [7,74,75]. This set of experts suggest that PET should be attenuation-corrected and performed not earlier than 3 weeks, preferably 6–8 weeks, after the last chemotherapy and 8–12 weeks after the end of external beam radiation or chemoradiotherapy. They find that visual assessment is adequate and propose to compare the ^{18}F-FDG uptake in residual masses $\geq$2 cm to the mediastinal blood pool activity. Activity of smaller masses or normal-size lymph nodes should not exceed surrounding background activity. Residual focal liver or spleen lesions should be considered positive if their uptake exceeds normal liver or spleen activity. Diffusely increased splenic uptake exceeding liver uptake should be considered positive unless the patient is on cytokines that might account for increased splenic uptake for at least 10 days. Diffusely increased bone marrow uptake is expected after chemotherapy, especially if assisted by cytokines. Clearly increased focal uptake may indicate residual bone marrow involvement. It is, however, recommended to compare the post-treatment PET with the pre-treatment study, if available, to check for bone marrow uptake and to compare the sites of uptake. In the presence of pre-treatment focal bone marrow involvement, post-treatment scans may have a patchy appearance due to the increased uptake in non-affected bone marrow adjacent to responding (negative) sites of lymphoma involvement. All these response definitions, however, leave space for quite an important grey zone.

Therefore, attempts have been made to further refine the interpretation of low to very low uptake. Measuring the reduction of SUV might have some advantage over visual interpretation for the evaluation of response to treatment [76]. With a cut-off value of 65.7% SUV reduction, 14 of 34 patients considered non-responders at visual analysis were reclassified as responders. After reclassification, PET non-responders had a 2-year event-free survival (EFS) estimate of 21%, whereas it was 51% in patients considered non-responders when relying on visual interpretation of PET.

Impact on Therapy of Interim 18F-FDG PET
All these publications are concordant in indicating the excellent prognostic value of interim ^{18}F-FDG PET in HL and NHL. It needs to be recognized, however, that the evidence of therapy changes based on the results of interim PET/CT, either in the sense of early introduction of intensification regimens or of reducing the prospected treatment, is still lacking. These questions are the object of several ongoing prospective trials, the results of which are eagerly expected. As yet, we do not know if early intensification of treatment in PET non-responders changes outcome or only increases toxicity. We also do not know if less treatment, such

as a reduced number of chemotherapy courses, allows quality of life improvement by sparing toxicity with similar outcome. Another question addresses the necessity and extent of consolidation radiotherapy, especially in young patients with HL. Could it be skipped or reduced without compromising outcome? And how will the results of ^{18}F-FDG PET influence radiation treatment planning? [77,78]

18F-FDG PET in the Evaluation of Stem Cell Transplantation
Several studies have addressed the question of the role of ^{18}F-FDG PET in association with autologous stem cell transplant (ASCT) in lymphoma [79,80]. Sixty consecutive lymphoma patients, who underwent consolidation by ASCT after achieving remission (31 complete, 23 partial), were studied.[81] In patients with negative ^{18}F-FDG PET before ASCT, the estimated 1-year EFS was 80% compared with 43% in patients who did not achieve ^{18}F-FDG negativity before ASCT. In patients who remained ^{18}F-FDG-positive on post-ASCT PET, 1-year EFS was only 25%. Multivariate analysis indicated that, independent of the histological subtype of lymphoma and timing of ASCT, the most important adverse prognostic factor was persistence of ^{18}F-FDG uptake on post-ASCT PET.

18F-FDG PET Monitoring Response to Treatment of Aggressive Hodgkin's Lymphoma and non-Hodgkin's Lymphoma
^{18}F-FDG PET/CT in assessing the response to treatment of aggressive HL and NHL and especially in identifying patients with low and high risk of relapse, already plays a role in the management of such patients [82]. Several studies are ongoing with the aim to determine if adapting treatment according to the results of early ^{18}F-FDG PET allows either to offer better outcome to patients with unfavorable prognosis at the expense of higher toxicity or to diminish cytotoxic treatment in those with low-risk disease while preserving favorable outcome. The results of these trials need to provide the evidence of the appropriateness of such changes in therapy before they can be introduced into the clinical management of patients with malignant lymphoma.

Guidelines and Recommendations for the Use of 18F-FDG PET and PET/CT in Lymphoma
The NCCN has incorporated ^{18}F-FDG PET in the evaluation and management algorithm of most HL and NHL [11]. The use of ^{18}F-FDG PET (PET/CT where available) is recommended in the following clinical scenarios: (1) baseline for lymphoma that are potentially curative (HD, DLBCL); (2) baseline to exclude systemic disease in clinically localized lymphoma (HD, DLBCL, FL, mantle cell, AIDS-related B-cell, nodal and splenic marginal zone, peripheral T cell, marginal B-cell lymphoma); (3) to evaluate residual masses; (4) to monitor therapy of aggressive lymphoma (HD, DLBCL). ^{18}F-FDG PET is not indicated: (1) to monitor therapy if CT is normal and (2) for surveillance.

Consensus recommendations regarding the use of ^{18}F-FDG PET for assessment response have been published by the imaging subcommittee of the IHP [7]: (1) pre-therapy ^{18}F-FDG PET imaging is strongly encouraged but not mandatory for aggressive lymphoma (HL, DLBCL, mantle cell lymphoma and FL) because they are routinely ^{18}F-FDG avid. However, pre-therapy ^{18}F-FDG

PET imaging is mandatory for lymphomas that are not typically ^{18}F-FDG avid, if response to treatment will also be evaluated with ^{18}F-FDG PET. (2) The timing of ^{18}F-FDG PET is critical to avoid equivocal interpretations. ^{18}F-FDG PET should be performed at least 3 weeks and preferably 6–8 weeks after completion of chemotherapy and 8–12 weeks after radiation therapy. For evaluation during therapy, ^{18}F-FDG PET imaging should be performed as close as possible before the subsequent cycle of therapy. (3) Visual assessment alone is adequate for interpreting PET findings as positive or negative. Mediastinal blood pool activity is used as a reference for assessment of residual masses greater than 2 cm. (4) Specific criteria for defining PET positivity in liver, spleen, lung and bone marrow are described in a previous section. (5) Treatment monitoring during the course of therapy should only be done in the setting of clinical trials.

In clinical trials, Cheson et al.[8] recommends the use of ^{18}F-FDG PET for potentially curable reliably ^{18}F-FDG-avid lymphomas (HL and DLBCL), including a pre-therapy PET and response assessment PET. However, for routinely ^{18}F-FDG-avid aggressive and indolent lymphomas that are incurable and for variably ^{18}F-FDG-avid lymphomas, a pre-therapy ^{18}F-FDG PET is recommended only if overall response rate (ORR) and CR are end points. If the pre-therapy PET is positive, PET is recommended to assess response to treatment. At mid-treatment, ^{18}F-FDG PET is recommended only in clinical trials.

The SNM procedure guidelines [4] and ACR practice guidelines [5] for tumor imaging using ^{18}F-FDG PET/CT address evaluation of malignancies in general. These procedure/practice guidelines include recommendations regarding preparation of the patient, protocols for PET and CT, reporting PET/CT and training of personnel who perform and interpret PET/CT. Regarding monitoring the response to therapy, the SNM procedure guidelines recommend a comparison of extent and intensity of uptake between the pre- and post-therapy images. A change of intensity of uptake with semi-quantitative measurements, expressed in absolute values and percent change, may be appropriate in some clinical scenarios. However, the technical protocol and analysis of images need to be consistent in the two sets of images. The impacts of radiotherapy on PET signals are described in greater detail in the chapters specifically dealing with those histologic subtypes.

REFERENCES

1. DA Podoloff, RH Advani, C Allred, et al. NCCN Task Force Report: positron emission tomography (PET/computed tomography (CT) scanning in cancer. J Natl Compr Canc Netw 5(Suppl 1):S1-22, 2007. www.nccn.org.

2. JW Fletcher, B Djulbegovic, HP Soares, et al. Recommendations for the use of FDG (fluorine-18, (2-[^{18}F]Fluoro-2-deoxy-D-glucose) positron emission tomography in oncology. J Nucl Med 49:480–508, 2008.

3. RE Coleman, D Delbeke, MJ Guiberteau, et al. Intersociety dialogue on concurrent PET-CT with an integrated imaging system: from the Joint ACR/SNM/SCBT-MR PET-CT Working Group. J Nucl Med 46:1225–39, 2005.

4. ACR Practice Guidelines for performing FDG PET/CT in oncology. www.ACR.org.

5. LK Shankar, JM Hoffman, S Bacharach, et al.; National Cancer Institute. Consensus recommendations for the use of 18F-FDG PET as an indicator of therapeutic response in patients in National Cancer Institute Trials. J Nucl Med 47(6):1059–66, 2006.

6. ME Juweid, S Stroobants, OS Hoekstra, et al. Use of positron emission tomography for response assessment of lymphoma: consensus of the Imaging Subcommittee of International Harmonization Project in Lymphoma. J Clin Oncol 25(5):571–78, 2007.

7. BD Cheson, B Pfistner, ME Juweid, et al. Revised response criteria for malignant lymphoma. J Clin Oncol 25(5):579–86, 2007.

8. GJR Cook, I Fogelman, MN Maisey. Normal physiological and benign pathological variants of 18-fluoro-2-deoxyglucose positron emission tomography scanning: potential for error in interpretation. Semin Nucl Med 26:308–14, 1996.

9. H Engel, H Steinert, A Buck, et al. Whole body PET: physiological and artifactual fluorodeoxyglucose accumulations. J Nucl Med 37:441–46, 1996.

10. SS Gambhir, J Czernin, J Schimmer, et al. A tabulated summary of the FDG PET literature. J Nucl Med 42(Suppl):1S–93S, 2001.

11. IF Ciernik, E Dizendorf, B Baumert, et al. Radiation treatment planning with an integrated positron emission and computer tomography (PET/CT): a feasibility study. Int J Radiation Biol Phys 57:853–63, 2003.

12. M Hutchings, A Loft, M Hansen, et al. Different histopathological subtypes of Hodgkin lymphoma show significantly different levels of FDG uptake. Hematol Oncol 24:146–50, 2006.

13. National Cancer Institute: http://www.cancer.gov/cancer-topics/.

14. NL Harris, ES Jaffe, J Diebold, et al. World Health Organization classification of neoplastic diseases of the hematopoietic and lymphoid tissues: report of the Clinical Advisory Committee meeting-Airlie House, Virginia, November 1997. J Clin Oncol 17:3835–49 (WHO), 1999.

15. Ping Lu. Staging and classification of lymphoma. Semin Nucl Med 35:160–64, 2005.

16. H Schoder, A Noy, M Gonen, et al. Intensity of 18fluorodeoxyglucose uptake in positron emission tomography distinguishes between indolent and aggressive non-Hodgkin's lymphoma. J Clin Oncol 23(21):4643–51, 2005.

17. R Elstrom, L Guan, G Baker, et al. Utility of FDG-PET scanning in lymphoma by WHO classification. Blood 101(10): 3875–76, 2003.

18. N Tsukamoto, M Kojima, M Hasegawa, et al. The usefulness of (18)F-fluorodeoxyglucose positron emission tomography ((18)F-FDG-PET) and a comparison of (18)F-FDG-pet with (67)gallium scintigraphy in the evaluation of lymphoma: relation to histologic subtypes based on the World Health Organization classification. Cancer 110(3):652–59, 2007.

19. L Brepoels, S Stroobants, W De Wever, et al. Positron emission tomography in mantle cell lymphoma. Leuk Lymphoma 49(9):1693–1701, 2008.

20. S Kako, K Izutsu, Y Ota, et al. T-cell FDG-PET in T-cell and NK-cell neoplasms. Ann Oncol 18:1685–90, 2007.

21. G Jerusalem, Y Beguin, F Najjar, et al. Positron emission tomography (PET) with 18F-fluorodeoxyglucose (18F-FDG) for the staging of low-grade non-Hodgkin's lymphoma (NHL). Ann Oncol 12:825–30, 2001.

22. JF Bruzzi, H Macapinlac, AM Tsimberidou, et al. Detection of Richter's transformation of chronic lymphocytic leukemia by PET/CT. J Nucl Med 47:1267–73, 2006.

23. F Najjar, R Hustinx, G Jerusalem, et al. Positron emission tomography (PET) for staging low-grade non-Hodgkin's lymphomas (NHL). Cancer Biother Radiopharm 16:297–304, 2001.

24. M Hoffmann, K Kletter, A Becherer, et al. 18F-fluorodeoxyglucose positron emission tomography (18F-FDG-PET) for staging and follow-up of marginal zone B-cell lymphoma. Oncology 64:336–40, 2003.

25. NA Mohile, LE Abrey. Primary central nervous system lymphoma. Neurol Clin 25(4):1193–1207, 2007.

26. SS Rosenfeld, JM Hoffman, RE Coleman, et al. Studies of primary central nervous system lymphoma with fluorine-18-fluorodeoxyglucose positron emission tomography. J Nucl Med 33:532–36, 1992.

27. AE Heald, JM Hoffman, JA Bartlett, et al. Differentiation of central nervous system lesions in AIDS patients using positron emission tomography (PET). J Int STD AIDS 7:337–46, 1996.

28. NA Mohile, LM Deangelis, LE Abrey. The utility of body FDG PET in staging primary central nervous system lymphoma. Neurol Oncol 10(2):223–28, 2008.

29. J Okada, H Oonishi, K Yoshikawa, et al. FDG-PET for predicting the prognosis of malignant lymphoma. Ann Nucl Med 8:187–91, 1994.

30. L Kostakoglu, SJ Goldsmith. Positron emission tomography in lymphoma: comparison with computed tomography and gallium-67 single photon emission computed tomography. Clin Lymph 1:67–74, 2000.

31. R Bar-Shalom, M Mor, N Yefremov, et al. The value of Ga-67 scintigraphy and F-18 fluorodeoxyglucose positron emission tomography in staging and monitoring the response of lymphoma to treatment. Semin Nucl Med 31:177–90, 2001.

32. O Israel, Z Keidar, R Bar-Shalom. Positron emission tomography in the evaluation of lymphoma. Semin Nucl Med 34:166–79, 2004.

33. P Seam, ME Juweid, BD Cheson. The role of FDG-PET scans in patients with lymphoma. Blood 110(10):3507–16, 2007.

34. I Buchmann, M Reinhardt, K Elsner, et al. 2-(fluorine-18) fluoro-2-deoxy-D-glucose positron emission tomography in the detection and staging of malignant lymphoma. A bicenter trial. Cancer 91(5):889–99, 2001.

35. CR Isasi, P Lu, MD Blaufox. A metaanalysis of 18F-2-deoxy-2-fluoro-D-glucose positron emission tomography in the staging and restaging of patients with lymphoma. Cancer 104(5):1066–74, 2005.

36. R Thill, J Neuerburg, U Fabry, et al. Comparison of findings with 18-FDG PET and CT in pretherapeutic staging of malignant lymphoma. Nuklearmedizin 36:234–39, 1997.

37. F Moog, M Bangerter, CG Diederichs, et al. Extranodal malignant lymphoma: detection with FDG PET versus CT. Radiology 206:475–81, 1998.

38. F Moog, M Bangerter, J Kotzerke, et al. 18-F-fluorodeoxyglucose-positron emission tomography as a new approach to detect lymphomatous bone marrow. J Clin Oncol 16: 603–9, 1998.

39. R Carr, SF Barrington, B Madan, et al. Detection of lymphoma in bone marrow by whole-body positron emission tomography. Blood 91:3340–46, 1998.

40. EE Pakos, AD Fotopoulos, JP Ioannidis. 18F-FDG PET for evaluation of bone marrow infiltration in staging of lymphoma: a meta-analysis. J Nucl Med 46(6):958–63, 2005.

41. LS Freudenberg, G Antoch, Schütt P, et al. FDG-PET/CT in re-staging of patients with lymphoma. Eur J Nucl Med Molec Imaging 31(3):325–29, 2004.

42. H Schöder, SM Larson, HW Yeung. PET/CT in oncology: integration into clinical management of lymphoma, melanoma, and gastrointestinal malignancies. J Nucl Med 45(Suppl):72S–81S, 2004.

43. NG Schaefer, TF Hany, C Taverna, et al. Non-Hodgkin lymphoma and Hodgkin disease: coregistered FDG PET and CT at staging and restaging–do we need contrast-enhanced CT? Radiology 232(3):823–29, 2004.

44. P Raanani, Y Shasha, C Perry, et al. Is CT scan still necessary for staging in Hodgkin and non-Hodgkin lymphoma patients in the PET/CT era? Ann Oncol 17(1):117–22, 2006.

45. B Rodríguez-Vigil, N Gómez-León, I Pinilla, et al. PET/CT in lymphoma: prospective study of enhanced full-dose PET/CT versus unenhanced low-dose PET/CT. J Nucl Med 47:1643–48, 2006.

46. RJ Hicks, MP Mac Manus, JF Seymour. Initial staging of lymphoma with positron emission tomography and computed tomography. Semin Nucl Med 35:165–75, 2005.

47. G Jerusalem, R Hustinx, Y Beguin, et al. Evaluation of therapy for lymphoma. Semin Nucl Med 35:186–96, 2005.

48. AK Buck, C Kratochwil, G Glatting, et al. Early assessment of therapy response in malignant lymphoma with the thymidine analogue [18F]FLT. Eur J Nucl Med Mol Imaging 34(11):1775–82, 2007.

49. A Iagaru, ML Goris, SS Gambhir. Perspectives of molecular imaging and radioimmunotherapy in lymphoma. Radiol Clin North Am 46(2):243–52, 2008.

50. M Bangerter, J Kotzerke, M Griesshammer, et al. Positron emission tomography with 18-fluorodeoxyglucose in the staging and follow-up of lymphoma in the chest. Acta Oncol 38(6):799–804, 1999.

51. K Spaepen, L Mortelmans. Evaluation of treatment response in patients with lymphoma using [18F]FDG-PET: differences between non-Hodgkin's lymphoma and Hodgkin's disease. Q J Nucl Med 45(3):269–73, 2001.

52. BD Cheson, SJ Horning, B Coiffier, et al. Report of an international workshop to standardize response criteria for non-Hodgkin's lymphomas. NCI Sponsored International Working Group. J Clin Oncol 17(4):1244, 1999.

53. ME Juweid, GA Wiseman, JM Vose, et al. Response assessment of aggressive non-Hodgkin's lymphoma by integrated International Workshop Criteria and fluorine-18-fluorodeoxyglucose positron emission tomography. J Clin Oncol 23(21):4652–61, 2005.

54. G Jerusalem, Y Beguin, MF Fassotte, et al. Whole-body positron emission tomography using 18F-fluorodeoxyglucose

for posttreatment evaluation in Hodgkin's disease and non-Hodgkin's lymphoma has higher diagnostic and prognostic value than classical computed tomography scan imaging. Blood 94(2):429–33, 1999.

55. NG Mikhaeel, AR Timothy, MJ O'Doherty, et al. 18-FDG-PET as a prognostic indicator in the treatment of aggressive Non-Hodgkin's lymphoma-comparison with CT. Leuk Lymphoma 39(5–6):543–53, 2000.

56. T Terasawa, T Nihashi, T Hotta, et al. 18F-FDG PET for posttherapy assessment of Hodgkin's disease and aggressive Non-Hodgkin's lymphoma: a systematic review. J Nucl Med 49(1):13–21, 2008.

57. L Kostakoglu, SJ Goldsmith, JP Leonard, et al. FDG-PET after 1 cycle of therapy predicts outcome in diffuse large cell lymphoma and classic Hodgkin disease. Cancer 107(11): 2678–87, 2006.

58. K Spaepen, S Stroobants, P Dupont, et al. Early restaging positron emission tomography with (18)F-fluorodeoxyglucose predicts outcome in patients with aggressive non-Hodgkin's lymphoma. Ann Oncol 13(9):1356–63, 2002.

59. NG Mikhaeel, M Hutchings, et al. FDG-PET after two to three cycles of chemotherapy predicts progression-free and overall survival in high-grade non-Hodgkin lymphoma. Ann Oncol 16(9):1514–23, 2005.

60. C Haioun, E Itti, A Rahmouni, et al. [18F]fluoro-2-deoxy-D-glucose positron emission tomography (FDG-PET) in aggressive lymphoma: an early prognostic tool for predicting patient outcome. Blood 106(4):1376–81, 2005.

61. A Gallamini, L Rigacci, F Merli, et al. The predictive value of positron emission tomography scanning performed after two courses of standard therapy on treatment outcome in advanced stage Hodgkin's disease. Haematologica 91(4):475–81, 2006.

62. M Hutchings, A Loft, M Hansen, et al. FDG-PET after two cycles of chemotherapy predicts treatment failure and progression-free survival in Hodgkin lymphoma. Blood 107(1):52–59, 2006.

63. JM Engles, SA Quarless, E Mambo, et al. Stunning and its effect on 3H-FDG uptake and key gene expression in breast cancer cells undergoing chemotherapy. J Nucl Med 47(4):603–8, 2006.

64. GJ Kelloff, DM Sullivan, W Wilson, et al. FDG-PET lymphoma demonstration project invitational workshop. Acad Radiol 14(3):330–39, 2007.

65. SM Larson, Y Erdi, T Akhurst, et al. Tumor treatment response based on visual and quantitative changes in global tumor glycolysis using PET-FDG imaging. The visual response score and the change in total lesion glycolysis. Clin Positron Imaging 2(3):159–71, 1999.

66. T Kazama, SC Faria, V Varavithya, et al. FDG PET in the evaluation of treatment for lymphoma: clinical usefulness and pitfalls. Radiographics 25(1):191–207, 2005.

67. HM Abdel-Dayem, G Rosen, H El-Zeftawy, et al. Fluorine-18 fluorodeoxyglucose splenic uptake from extramedullary hematopoiesis after granulocyte colony-stimulating factor stimulation. Clin Nucl Med 24:319–22, 1999.

68. S Gundlapalli, B Ojha, JM Mountz. Granulocyte colony-stimulating factor: confounding F-18 FDG uptake in outpatient positron emission tomographic facilities for patients receiving ongoing treatment of lymphoma. Clin Nucl Med 27:140–41, 2002.

69. B Ferdinand, P Gupta, EL Kramer. Spectrum of thymic uptake at 18F-FDG PET. Radiographics 24:1611–16, 2004.

70. M Baudard, F Comte, AM Conge, et al. Importance of [18F] fluorodeoxyglucose-positron emission tomography scanning for the monitoring of responses to immunotherapy in follicular lymphoma. Leuk Lymphoma 48(2):381–88, 2007.

71. JE Wooldridge. Can a positive positron emission tomography scan be positive news? Leuk Lymphoma 48(2):227–28, 2007.

72. JM Joyce, B Degirmenci, S Jacobs, et al. FDG PET CT assessment of treatment response after yttrium-90 ibritumomab tiuxetan radioimmunotherapy. Clin Nucl Med 30(8):564–68, 2005.

73. PL Zinzani, M Tani, S Fanti, et al. A phase II trial of CHOP chemotherapy followed by yttrium 90 ibritumomab tiuxetan (Zevalin) for previously untreated elderly diffuse large B-cell lymphoma patients. Ann Oncol 19(4):769–73, 2008.

74. L Brepoels, S Stroobants, W De Wever, et al. Hodgkin lymphoma: response assessment by revised International Workshop Criteria. Leuk Lymphoma 48(8):1539–47, 2007.

75. L Brepoels, S Stroobants, W De Wever, et al. Aggressive and indolent non-Hodgkin's lymphoma: response assessment by integrated international workshop criteria. Leuk Lymphoma 48(8):1522–30, 2007.

76. C Lin, E Itti, C Haioun, et al. Early 18F-FDG PET for prediction of prognosis in patients with diffuse large B-cell lymphoma: SUV-based assessment versus visual analysis. J Nucl Med 48(10):1626–32, 2007.

77. L Specht. 2-[18F]Fluoro-2-deoxyglucose positron-emission tomography in staging, response evaluation, and treatment planning of lymphomas. Semin Radiat Oncol 17:190–97, 2007.

78. ST Kahn, C Flowers, MJ Lechowicz, et al. Value of PET restaging after chemotherapy for non-Hodgkin's lymphoma: implications for consolidation radiotherapy. Int J Radiat Oncol Biol Phys 66(4):961–65, 2006.

79. PB Johnston, GA Wiseman, IN Micallef. Positron emission tomography using F-18 fluorodeoxyglucose pre- and post-autologous stem cell transplant in non-Hodgkin's lymphoma. Bone Marrow Trans 41(11):919–25, 2008.

80. BW Schot, JM Zijlstra, WJ Sluiter, et al. Early FDG-PET assessment in combination with clinical risk scores determines prognosis in recurring lymphoma. Blood 109(2):486–91, 2007.

81. JE Filmont, C Gisselbrecht, X Cuenca, et al. The impact of pre- and post-transplantation positron emission tomography using 18-fluorodeoxyglucose on poor-prognosis lymphoma patients undergoing autologous stem cell transplantation. Cancer 110(6):1361–99, 2007.

82. YL Kasamon, RJ Jones, RL Wahl. Integrating PET and PET/CT into the risk-adapted therapy of lymphoma. J Nucl Med 48(Suppl 1):19S–27S, 2007.

3   Positron Emission Tomography/Computed Tomography in Radiotherapy Treatment Planning

Stephanie A Terezakis and Joachim Yahalom

Introduction

Positron emission tomography (PET) using 2-[18F] fluoro-2-deoxyglucose (FDG) has been increasingly utilized as a diagnostic tool in lymphoma management. FDG is a radiolabeled analog of glucose and FDG-PET is a functional imaging modality that is based on the premise that tumor cells utilize increased amounts of glucose relative to normal cells. Therefore, FDG accumulates within tumor cells and gamma rays, which are emitted indirectly, are detected. Images can then be reconstructed in a three-dimensional (3D) fashion. FDG-PET is now accepted as a standard component of staging and treatment response evaluation for lymphoma patients. Owing to the utility of FDG-PET, interest in incorporating its use in radiation treatment planning has grown.

Staging of lymphoma is accomplished using physical examination, tissue biopsy including bone marrow biopsy, and imaging modalities. The advent of computed tomography (CT) has allowed for greater anatomic definition and led to improvements in initial disease staging and assessment of treatment response. In addition, CT imaging has enhanced accurate delineation of radiation treatment fields. However, CT has its limitations. In the absence of frank lymphadenopathy, small volume nodal disease can be missed. Conversely, residual scarring and bulky soft tissue masses that linger radiographically despite a complete treatment response can obscure evaluation. Therefore, PET has become an important complementary tool for evaluating disease extent in lymphoma patients.

Positron Emission Tomography/Computed Tomography Utility in Staging

PET/CT has become a standard imaging tool for lymphoma staging, as multiple studies have shown that FDG-PET has increased sensitivity and specificity compared to CT scan alone [1–7]. For example, Stumpe et al. demonstrated a specificity of only 41% for CT scan in staging Hodgkin's disease (HD) patients, but a specificity of 96% for FDG-PET. Similarly for non-Hodgkin's lymphoma (NHL) patients, FDG-PET had a specificity of 100% and CT scan had a specificity of merely 67% [5]. In a study by Schoder et al., PET altered the clinical stage in 46% of patients, resulting in change of management for 42% of patients studied [4].

FDG-PET frequently results in the upstaging of lymphoma patients and therefore, management decisions may change once PET information is obtained [8]. For example, patients with advanced-stage disease may not be candidates for combined modality therapy and may receive chemotherapy alone (see Fig. 3.1). It is widely presumed that the addition of FDG-PET diagnostic information will ultimately lead to better clinical outcomes. However, FDG-PET is not necessarily useful for all lymphoma subtypes. Abnormal FDG uptake has been found to correlate with proliferative activity and malignancy grade because of the enhanced metabolic activity of tumor cells [4,8–11]. Aggressive

NHL such as diffuse large B-cell lymphoma as well as HD are more likely to be FDG avid as compared to indolent lymphomas, such as follicular and marginal zone types. Studies have demonstrated widely variable FDG avidity in low-grade lymphomas, suggesting that PET may not be as helpful in this setting [12–16].

The difficulty with deriving staging conclusions from FDG-PET lies in our inability to obtain pathologic proof of disease at each FDG-avid disease site. It is commonly known that FDG avidity may be due to inflammation, infection and reactivity rather than malignancy. However, it is unfortunately impractical to subject patients to innumerable procedures particularly considering the systemic nature of lymphomatous disease. Therefore, physicians must continue to integrate multiple sources of staging information, including FDG-PET scan, CT scan, physical examination and laboratory testing, to make treatment recommendations.

Positron Emission Tomography/Computed Tomography Utility in Treatment Response

FDG-PET is also routinely used to assess treatment response both during and after therapy. CT scan is frequently obtained, but the appearance of a residual mass is a common occurrence. Formal criteria to assess response based on the size of a mass on post-treatment CT scan have been created, but residual masses often represent scarring or necrosis that cannot be effectively discerned from viable disease on CT scan. FDG-PET can help determine whether a residual mass represents active disease. The International Working Group (IWG) has incorporated FDG-PET information in establishing treatment response criteria for both HD and NHL. Complete remission (CR) may be achieved in patients with either a pre-treatment positive PET scan or without a pre-treatment PET if there is a post-treatment residual mass of any size as long as it is PET negative [17–19].

After a given number of chemotherapy cycles, FDG-PET is acquired to assess whether a particular systemic therapy is effective. FDG-PET is also obtained in routine follow-up after treatment has been completed. Multiple studies have demonstrated that positive PET findings are highly predictive for relapse after completion of standard therapy [20–25]. There is significant interest in determining whether treatment modifications should be based on FDG-PET scan response early in a patient's chemotherapy course. In a study by Picardi et al., 260 patients with bulky HD were treated with induction chemotherapy and 160 achieved a negative PET. They were subsequently randomized to receive either further treatment with radiation or observation. After a median follow-up of 40 months, 14% of patients treated with chemotherapy alone had histologic confirmation of malignant disease as compared to 4% of patients in the radiotherapy arm. All patients with relapse in the chemotherapy group were found to have malignant disease within the bulky or contiguous nodal region [26]. Thus, although patients have a negative PET, they may

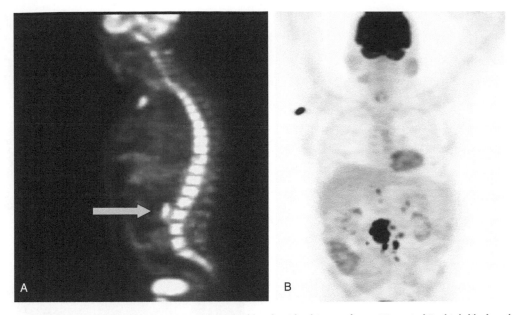

Figure 3.1 Staging impact with PET/CT simulation. This patient was a 70-year-old male with a history of stage III atypical Burkitt's-like lymphoma, who presented for involved-field radiation prior to stem cell transplantation to a site of residual retroperitoneal lymphadenopathy. FDG uptake is demonstrated on the pre-simulation PET scan shown in the first figure at the site of the arrow. He presented 2 weeks after his initial PET scan for PET/CT simulation. The second figure demonstrates progression of disease in the abdominal and pelvic regions noted at the time of simulation. Management plans to proceed with radiation were aborted and the patient returned for further chemotherapy. Patients with aggressive lymphomas may benefit from PET/CT simulation even when they have had a recent PET because of the potential for rapid progression of disease.

still harbor microscopic residual disease. Therefore, an element of standard treatment cannot be omitted until we better understand the role of PET in the evaluation of treatment response.

Further studies are clearly warranted to define the role of PET in the assessment of treatment response. A randomized trial designed by EORTC-GELA has recently opened for stage I–II HD patients to evaluate this controversy. In HD10, favorable patients will receive three courses of ABVD (adriamycin, bleomycin, vinblastine, dacarbazine) and involved-field radiotherapy (IFRT) with 30 Gy on the standard arm, while the experimental patients will be evaluated with PET after two courses of ABVD. If the patient is PET negative, they will receive a third cycle of ABVD without IFRT. Unfavorable patients will be studied in HD11, where the experimental design is the same but treatment consists of four courses of ABVD rather than three. The clinical outcomes of this study are eagerly awaited to better understand if treatment modifications can be made based on early interim PET scan results.

Positron Emission Tomography/Computed Tomography Role in Radiation Treatment Planning

CT scan simulation is a standard radiation planning tool that allows physicians to define the anatomic extent of a tumor as well as normal structures. Contouring on a CT radiation planning scan allows the physician to confidently define the involved-nodal treatment field(s) and delineate a tumor volume that can be treated conformally with advanced planning techniques. PET is particularly useful in lymphoma to define the extent of a patient's disease, therefore, PET information is often used to help design radiation treatment fields. To facilitate radiation treatment planning, an FDG-PET scan obtained in a nuclear medicine department can be co-registered to a CT treatment planning scan obtained in a department of radiation oncology. In these situations, the patient

can be placed in the treatment planning position using an appropriate immobilization device. The FDG-PET scan is then transferred and fused with the CT treatment planning scan. However, co-registration may be difficult if the patient's position varies between the two scans. With the introduction of dedicated PET/CT scanners for simulation, images can be acquired simultaneously and information derived from the FDG-PET portion of the scan can be immediately co-registered for use in tumor volume delineation (see Fig. 3.2).

The integration of FDG-PET in radiation treatment planning has been studied most extensively in patients with non-small cell lung cancer (NSCLC) and head and neck cancers, but studies examining target volume definition in lymphoma are scarce. Based on studies in NSCLC and head and neck, we have learned that information obtained at the time of FDG-PET simulation can result in significant changes in staging, management and target volumes. For example, in a study by Bradley et al., PET scan altered staging in 31% (8/26) of NSCLC patients [27]. TNM and AJCC staging also changed in 36 and 14% of head and neck patients, respectively, resulting in a change in the management of 25% of patients in a study by Koshy et al. [28]. The management of 23% of patients was altered from definitive to palliative based on information obtained at the time of PET simulation in a prospective study by Mah et al. [29].

Multiple studies investigating the impact of FDG-PET simulation in NSCLC and head and neck have also suggested that tumor volumes are altered when PET information is integrated into radiation planning [27,29–33]. In the study by Mah et al., three independent physicians who contoured target volumes would have had a geographic miss in 17–29% of cases using CT alone. A reduction in planning target volume (PTV) occurred in 24–70% of cases, while an increase in PTV occurred in 30–76% of cases

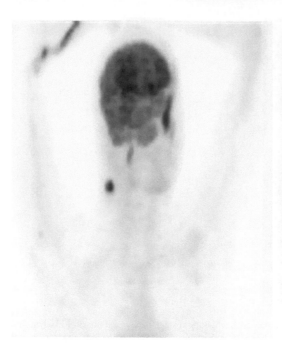
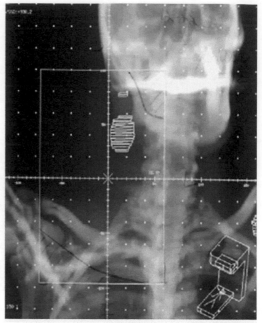

Figure 3.2 PET/CT simulation in implementation of IFRT. This patient was a 65-year-old male with refractory diffuse large B-cell lymphoma presenting for involved-field radiation to the right side of the neck. The right neck mass was easily identified on PET scan, but not clearly delineated on CT imaging. The patient underwent PET/CT simulation in the treatment position and the treatment field was designed using IFRT guidelines.

with the use of PET simulation [29]. Additional studies examining the change in PTV volume for NSCLC patients found an overall decrease in gross tumor volume (GTV) with the use of PET, while the study by Bradley et al. found no difference in tumor volume with the addition of PET [27,30,32]. An overall decrease in GTV was noted with the use of PET radiation planning for head and neck cancer patients as compared to tumor volumes delineated based on CT alone [34–37]. Two studies demonstrated no difference in tumor volumes for head and neck patients planned with PET simulation [38,39]. Although the integration of PET has clearly altered target volumes in multiple studies, no consistent trends have emerged and without pathology, we cannot know which tumor volume represents the true extent of disease. Only one study has attempted to correlate contoured tumor volumes with pathology. Daisne et al. examined surgical specimens of head and neck patients and found that PET was the most accurate modality to assess the true tumor volume [34].

The impact of FDG-PET integration in radiation treatment planning for lymphoma patients is an area under current active investigation. Initial studies performed have suggested that PET radiation planning will result in changes in target volume definition and may impact doses to normal structures. Lee et al. retrospectively assessed tumor volume definition in thoracic lymphoma patients by manually registering PET to a CT scan [40]. Ten positive PET scans were identified. In four of ten cases, the difference in lateral field extension of the treatment field was greater than 3.0 cm and in three of these cases, the PET-defined GTV was smaller than the GTV on CT scan. In two cases, the inferior extent of the AP/PA fields delineated was 12.0 and 14.4 cm greater with CT alone as compared to PET. Phantom planning demonstrated a decrease in lung dose by 50% when PET was utilized. By targeting the active site(s) of disease using PET information, doses to normal structures may be reduced.

In the study by Lee et al., the apparent CT scan abnormality was not completely included within the treatment field as the GTV was defined with PET information [40]. As demonstrated in the study by Picardi et al., patients with residual CT scan abnormality and a negative PET may continue to harbor malignant cells on a microscopic level [26]. At this time, we continue to include the entirety of the abnormality seen on CT scan, as there is no clear evidence to suggest that microscopic disease does not exist in sites that are PET negative (see Fig. 3.3). As studies correlating pathology with PET scan findings in lymphoma do not exist, we recommend an integrated approach to delineate tumor volumes by including abnormalities seen on both PET and CT scan.

Additional studies have been performed suggesting that PET radiation planning can result in a change in management and tumor volume definition for lymphoma patients, although the patient numbers in these investigations are small. Hutchings et al. recently studied 30 patients who received a staging FDG-PET/CT after a short course of ABVD and prior to radiation treatment for early-stage HD. IFRT planning was initially performed using a CT treatment planning scan alone, but patients were subsequently planned using an integrated PET/CT for contouring. The use of FDG-PET information would have resulted in an increase in the treated volume in seven patients and in these patients the volume receiving 90% of the prescription dose was increased by 8–87%. A decrease in the treated volume would have occurred in two patients, while the tumor volume remained the same in 20 patients [41]. A study by Dizendorf et al. reviewed the records of 202 consecutive patients who presented with various malignancies and underwent FDG-PET scan for the purpose of radiation treatment planning. Of this patient cohort, 24 were diagnosed with malignant lymphoma. After the integration of a pre-radiation PET scan, management strategy was altered in 21% of patients and a change in target volume was implemented in 13% of

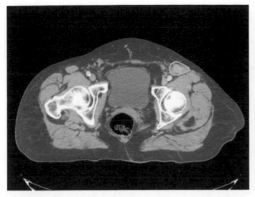
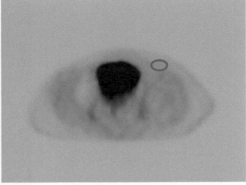

Figure 3.3 PET/CT simulation for staging and treatment planning in low-grade lymphoma. The patient was a 54-year-old female presenting with a left inguinal mass that was a biopsy-proven stage I low-grade follicular lymphoma. The mass is clearly delineated on CT scan as above. The patient had no recent PET scan. A PET/CT simulation was performed for both staging and treatment planning purposes. The PET was negative, which is not uncommon for low-grade lymphomas. The mass was contoured on CT and the patient was treated with involved-field radiation to the left inguinal region as per IFRT guidelines.

lymphoma patients [42]. Brianzoni et al. also studied 28 patients with a spectrum of malignancies of which four presented with NHL. FDG-PET scan was acquired in all patients and registered to CT images for radiation planning. Radiation treatment did not proceed in one patient because of findings on PET, although clinical target volume (CTV) was not altered in any of the patients in this small cohort [43].

In a recent study presented by our institution, 29 patients with 30 positive PET/CT treatment planning scans were analyzed retrospectively. Twenty-two patients underwent dedicated PET/CT simulation, while the remaining patients underwent a PET scan in the treatment position, which was subsequently fused to the CT treatment planning scan. Thirty-three treatment sites were re-contoured on both the CT scan alone as well as on the PET/CT fusion planning scan. Multiple anatomic sites as well as lymphoma subtypes were included. All patients were re-planned using both the volumes delineated on the CT and PET/CT treatment planning scans. A change in staging as well as management occurred in

7% (2/29) of patients. Ten percent of patients were treated to an increased number of treatment sites as a result of PET/CT planning. The GTV increased in 47% (15/32), decreased in 25% (8/32) and remained the same in 28% (9/32) of volumes delineated. The D95 and V95 decreased greater than 5% in six patients when the CT plan was used to the cover the PET volume. If it is assumed that the volume delineated using the integrated PET represents the site of active disease, these patients would not have had adequate coverage of their tumor volume had the CT treatment planning scan been used without the PET obtained at the time of simulation [44].

FDG-PET can clearly impact radiation field design and may result in dosimetric changes to both the tumor volume and normal structures (see Figs. 3.5 and 3.6). However, the study of PET integration in radiation planning for lymphoma remains under active investigation as patient numbers are small and definitive conclusions cannot yet be drawn. Although definitive guidelines do not exist, PET is now being actively used to define target volumes.

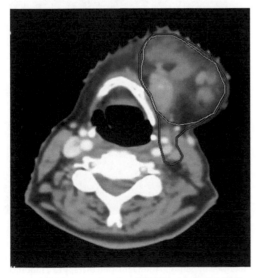
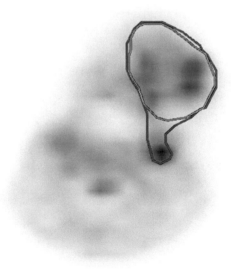

Figure 3.4 Incorporating a second treatment site after PET/CT simulation. This patient was an 82-year-old woman with diffuse large B-cell lymphoma who presented with a submandibular mass. The GTV contoured based on CT simulation alone is outlined in yellow, while the GTV contoured using PET/CT simulation is outlined in pink. An additional site was included in the GTV after PET/CT simulation when an ipsilateral cervical lymph node was FDG avid, although it was not enlarged by radiographic criteria.

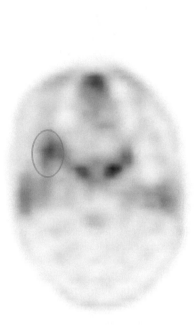
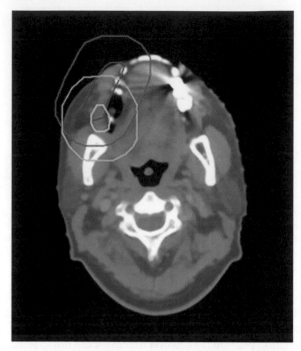

Figure 3.5 PET/CT simulation in target volume definition for IMRT. The patient was a 45-year-old man with relapsed stage I follicular lymphoma with a destructive lesion at the mandible. Owing to significant local inflammation, the lesion was difficult to localize on CT scan and the extent of the lesion was better defined with the addition of PET information. The GTV and PTV (red and pink, respectively) on CT scan alone were compared with the GTV and PTV (green and orange, respectively) when PET information from simulation was integrated. In this case, PET integration aided in delineating the target accurately, which is of utmost importance when creating a conformal plan for treatment.

Positron Emission Tomography/Computed Tomography Contribution in Radiation Field Design

Lymphoma management has evolved from the delivery of extended field radiation to the approach of combined modality therapy with involved-field lymph node irradiation (IFRT). Retrospective studies have suggested a decrease in second malignancy rate with IFRT as compared to extended field radiation [45–47]. Smaller treatment fields would also potentially impact on long-term toxicity by reducing cardiovascular disease. As fields have decreased in size, target volume definition has become an increasingly important dilemma for the radiation oncologist to ensure accuracy of the tumor volume. The advent of conformal techniques including 3D-conformal radiation treatment (3D-CRT) and intensity modulated radiotherapy (IMRT) has also placed the onus on the treating physician to precisely outline the treatment volume (see Fig. 3.7) [48].

Owing to the wide variability of involved-field definitions and prescribed doses amongst treating physicians, a need for clinical

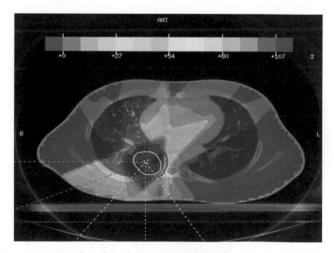

Figure 3.7 Dose conformality achieved using IMRT with guidance of PET/CT simulation for treatment volume definition. The patient was a 26-year-old male with refractory classical Hodgkin's lymphoma, who was initially treated with ABVD×6 followed by consolidation radiation therapy to a modified mantle field to 3600 cGy. He relapsed and presented with refractory disease in the right posterior lung. With the use of IMRT and enhancement of target volume definition with PET/CT simulation, it was feasible to re-treat a limited field encompassing the site of refractory disease to an additional dose of 3600 cGy.

Figure 3.6 IMRT after PET/CT simulation. The conformal plan created with IMRT for treatment demonstrating PTV coverage with the 100% isodose curve (yellow).

guidelines to define field borders has emerged [49]. The suggested guidelines created for the Cancer and Leukemia Group B (CALGB) studies in HD are now routinely used for delineating treatment fields. In designing a radiation treatment field using these principles, a lymph node region treated with IFRT is limited to the site of the clinically involved lymph node group based on Ann Arbor classification. The lymph node regions mainly involved include the unilateral neck, mediastinum and supraclavicular nodes, axilla including the supraclavicular and infraclavicular nodes, spleen, para-aortic lymph nodes and inguinal lymph nodes. The organ alone is treated when lymphoma presents in an extranodal site without lymph node involvement. The pre-chemotherapy volume is used for design of the treatment fields except at the transverse extent of the tumor when the post-chemotherapy volume is used. By limiting the transverse extent of the tumor volume, normal tissue can be spared. Both pre-chemotherapy and post-chemotherapy diagnostic information and imaging is critical for treatment field design.

In the management of early-stage HD, patients are often initially treated with chemotherapy followed by radiation. The post-chemotherapy PET scan is frequently negative in these cases. A PET/CT simulation can be acquired in patients who present after initial treatment with chemotherapy for evaluation of treatment response and for the purpose of treatment planning. When the post-chemotherapy PET is negative, the treatment field is based on the CT scan findings alone. However, treatment volumes continue to evolve, with recent data suggesting that patients treated with chemotherapy alone for early-stage HD, most frequently relapse in the initially involved lymph node(s) [26,50]. As a result, the EORTC-GELA have introduced the concept of involved-node radiation treatment (INRT), which entails delineating a CTV that includes the original pre-chemotherapy involved lymph node(s) [51]. The CTV is expanded by a 1-cm margin to create the PTV.

Girinsky et al. addressed the challenge of contouring the pre-chemotherapy volume using a post-chemotherapy PET/CT planning scan. The pre-treatment CT and FDG-PET scans performed in the treatment position were co-registered with a post-chemotherapy CT simulation planning scan in early-stage HD patients. FDG-PET helped to delineate lymph nodes that were otherwise undetectable on CT scan in 36% of patients. To apply the INRT concept, pre-chemotherapy FDG-PET information is invaluable to recognize sites of disease that require consolidative radiation [52]. Pre-chemotherapy PET scans are obtained on all patients who present prior to initial therapy at our institution and are utilized in designing post-chemotherapy treatment fields.

Positron Emission Tomography/Computed Tomography Limitations

PET/CT radiation planning can clearly enhance the accuracy of target volume delineation. However, there are multiple factors that can influence FDG uptake and PET interpretation. Windowing level, image resolution and patient motion, particularly during respiration, may affect the reproducibility of PET images. A standardized uptake value (SUV) threshold to define malignant versus benign tissue remains undefined in lymphoma patients. Some advocate defining FDG-avid areas as a percentage of intensity level relative to the maximum intensity. At our institution, each PET obtained at simulation is a full diagnostic scan. The

window level for contouring is matched to the window level used for diagnostic interpretation as defined by a nuclear medicine physician to standardize the definition of the GTV for radiation planning.

Another source of variation in PET imaging results when patients are prepared for their scan in a different manner because the time between tracer injection and scanning, patient blood glucose level, lesion size and scanning room temperature may all affect the measurement of FDG uptake. PET is an important complement to additional available information, including CT, physical examination and accessible pathology, and should be used within the proper clinical context. Due to the many factors that may affect PET results, clinical judgment is ultimately required to define the gross tumor. PET interpretation should also be performed in conjunction with a trained nuclear medicine physician to facilitate precise tumor volume definition.

Conclusions

FDG-PET plays an integral role in the management of lymphoma for staging, treatment response and radiation treatment planning. Multiple studies have suggested the advantage of the addition of PET to CT radiation planning scans for the treatment of various malignancies including lymphoma. The changes in target volume that occur with the integration of FDG-PET may potentially avoid a marginal miss or decrease the dose to surrounding normal structures. FDG-PET obtained at the time of simulation may also lead to changes in management. However, data defining the impact of FDG-PET in radiation planning of lymphoma remains scarce. Lymphoma radiation treatment fields shrink further because of the incorporation of IFRT and INRT concepts and the approach to radiation treatment has also become more conformal with the advent of IMRT. Therefore, the importance of accurately defining tumor volume has become remarkably apparent. PET/CT integration in radiation treatment planning is an area under active investigation and there are no current definitive guidelines on how to incorporate PET information. Thus, target volumes must be defined using information derived from FDG-PET, CT scan and clinical examination. Studies are eagerly awaited to further define the role of FDG-PET in radiation treatment planning for lymphoma patients.

REFERENCES

1. G Jerusalem, Y Beguin, MF Fassotte, et al. Whole-body positron emission tomography using 18F-fluorodeoxyglucose compared to standard procedures for staging patients with Hodgkin's disease. Haematologica 86:266–73, 2001.
2. M Sasaki, Y Kuwabara, H Koga, et al. Clinical impact of whole body FDG-PET on the staging and therapeutic decision making for malignant lymphoma. Ann Nucl Med 16:337–45, 2002.
3. C Schiepers, JE Filmont, J Czernin. PET for staging of Hodgkin's disease and non-Hodgkin's lymphoma. Eur J Nucl Med Mol Imaging 30(Suppl 1):S82–88, 2003.
4. H Schoder, J Meta, C Yap, et al. Effect of whole-body (18)F-FDG PET imaging on clinical staging and management of patients with malignant lymphoma. J Nucl Med 42:1139–43, 2001.
5. KD Stumpe, M Urbinelli, HC Steinert, et al. Whole-body positron emission tomography using fluorodeoxyglucose for staging of lymphoma: effectiveness and comparison with computed tomography. Eur J Nucl Med 25:721–28, 1998.

6. MR Weihrauch, D Re, S Bischoff, et al. Whole-body positron emission tomography using 18F-fluorodeoxyglucose for initial staging of patients with Hodgkin's disease. Ann Hematol 81:20–25, 2002.

7. A Wirth, JF Seymour, RJ Hicks, et al. Fluorine-18 fluorodeoxyglucose positron emission tomography, gallium-67 scintigraphy, and conventional staging for Hodgkin's disease and non-Hodgkin's lymphoma. Am J Med 112:262–68, 2002.

8. M Hutchings, A Loft, M Hansen, et al. Different histopathological subtypes of Hodgkin lymphoma show significantly different levels of FDG uptake. Hematol Oncol 24:146–50, 2006.

9. JS Newman, IR Francis, MS Kaminski, et al. Imaging of lymphoma with PET with 2-[F-18]-fluoro-2-deoxy-D-glucose: correlation with CT. Radiology 190:111–16, 1994.

10. J Okada, K Yoshikawa, K Imazeki, et al. The use of FDG-PET in the detection and management of malignant lymphoma: correlation of uptake with prognosis. J Nucl Med 32:686–91, 1991.

11. J Okada, K Yoshikawa, M Itami, et al. Positron emission tomography using fluorine-18-fluorodeoxyglucose in malignant lymphoma: a comparison with proliferative activity. J Nucl Med 33:325–29, 1992.

12. M Hoffmann, K Kletter, A Becherer, et al. 18F-fluorodeoxyglucose positron emission tomography (18F-FDG-PET) for staging and follow-up of marginal zone B-cell lymphoma. Oncology 64:336–40, 2003.

13. G Jerusalem, Y Beguin, F Najjar, et al. Positron emission tomography (PET) with 18F-fluorodeoxyglucose (18F-FDG) for the staging of low-grade non-Hodgkin's lymphoma (NHL). Ann Oncol 12:825–30, 2001.

14. F Najjar, R Hustinx, G Jerusalem, et al. Positron emission tomography (PET) for staging low-grade non-Hodgkin's lymphomas (NHL). Cancer Biother Radiopharm 16:297–304, 2001.

15. H Schoder, A Noy, M Gonen, et al. Intensity of 18fluorodeoxyglucose uptake in positron emission tomography distinguishes between indolent and aggressive non-Hodgkin's lymphoma. J Clin Oncol 23:4643–51, 2005.

16. S Wohrer, U Jaeger, K Kletter, et al. 18F-fluoro-deoxyglucose positron emission tomography (18F-FDG-PET) visualizes follicular lymphoma irrespective of grading. Ann Oncol 17:780–84, 2006.

17. BD Cheson, SJ Horning, B Coiffier, et al. Report of an international workshop to standardize response criteria for non-Hodgkin's lymphomas. NCI Sponsored International Working Group. J Clin Oncol 17:1244, 1999.

18. BD Cheson, B Pfistner, ME Juweid, et al. Revised response criteria for malignant lymphoma. J Clin Oncol 25:579–86, 2007.

19. ME Juweid, S Stroobants, OS Hoekstra, et al. Use of positron emission tomography for response assessment of lymphoma: consensus of the Imaging Subcommittee of International Harmonization Project in Lymphoma. J Clin Oncol 25:571–78, 2007.

20. A Gallamini, M Hutchings, L Rigacci, et al. Early interim 2-[18F]fluoro-2-deoxy-D-glucose positron emission tomography is prognostically superior to international prognostic score in advanced-stage Hodgkin's lymphoma: a report from a joint Italian-Danish study. J Clin Oncol 25:3746–52, 2007.

21. G Jerusalem, Y Beguin, MF Fassotte, et al. Whole-body positron emission tomography using 18F-fluorodeoxyglucose for posttreatment evaluation in Hodgkin's disease and non-Hodgkin's lymphoma has higher diagnostic and prognostic value than classical computed tomography scan imaging. Blood 94:429–33, 1999.

22. NG Mikhaeel, AR Timothy, O'MJ Doherty, et al. 18-FDG-PET as a prognostic indicator in the treatment of aggressive non-Hodgkin's lymphoma-comparison with CT. Leuk Lymphoma 39:543–53, 2000.

23. K Spaepen, S Stroobants, P Dupont, et al. Prognostic value of positron emission tomography (PET) with fluorine-18 fluorodeoxyglucose ([18F]FDG) after first-line chemotherapy in non-Hodgkin's lymphoma: is [18F]FDG-PET a valid alternative to conventional diagnostic methods? J Clin Oncol 19:414–19, 2001.

24. MR Weihrauch, D Re, K Scheidhauer, et al. Thoracic positron emission tomography using 18F-fluorodeoxyglucose for the evaluation of residual mediastinal Hodgkin disease. Blood 98:2930–34, 2001.

25. PL Zinzani, G Musuraca, L Alinari, et al. Predictive role of positron emission tomography in the outcome of patients with follicular lymphoma. Clin Lymphoma Myeloma 7:291–95, 2007.

26. M Picardi, De A Renzo, F Pane, et al. Randomized comparison of consolidation radiation versus observation in bulky Hodgkin's lymphoma with post-chemotherapy negative positron emission tomography scans. Leuk Lymphoma 48:1721–27, 2007.

27. J Bradley, WL Thorstad, S Mutic, et al. Impact of FDG-PET on radiation therapy volume delineation in non-small-cell lung cancer. Int J Radiat Oncol Biol Phys 59:78–86, 2004.

28. M Koshy, AC Paulino, R Howell, et al. F-18 FDG PET-CT fusion in radiotherapy treatment planning for head and neck cancer. Head Neck 27:494–502, 2005.

29. K Mah, CB Caldwell, YC Ung, et al. The impact of (18) FDG-PET on target and critical organs in CT-based treatment planning of patients with poorly defined non-small-cell lung carcinoma: a prospective study. Int J Radiat Oncol Biol Phys 52:339–50, 2002.

30. IF Ciernik, E Dizendorf, BG Baumert, et al. Radiation treatment planning with an integrated positron emission and computer tomography (PET/CT): a feasibility study. Int J Radiat Oncol Biol Phys 57:853–63, 2003.

31. YE Erdi, K Rosenzweig, AK Erdi, et al. Radiotherapy treatment planning for patients with non-small cell lung cancer using positron emission tomography (PET). Radiother Oncol 62:51–60, 2002.

32. A van Der Wel, S Nijsten, M Hochstenbag, et al. Increased therapeutic ratio by 18FDG-PET CT planning in patients with clinical CT stage N2-N3M0 non-small-cell lung cancer: a modeling study. Int J Radiat Oncol Biol Phys 61:649–55, 2005.

33. LJ Vanuytsel, JF Vansteenkiste, SG Stroobants, et al. The impact of (18)F-fluoro-2-deoxy-D-glucose positron emission tomography (FDG-PET) lymph node staging on the radiation treatment volumes in patients with non-small cell lung cancer. Radiother Oncol 55:317–24, 2000.

34. JF Daisne, T Duprez, B Weynand, et al. Tumor volume in pharyngolaryngeal squamous cell carcinoma: comparison at CT, MR imaging, and FDG PET and validation with surgical specimen. Radiology 233:93–100, 2004.

35. DE Heron, RS Andrade, J Flickinger, et al. Hybrid PET-CT simulation for radiation treatment planning in head-and-neck cancers: a brief technical report. Int J Radiat Oncol Biol Phys 60:1419–24, 2004.

36. AC Paulino, M Koshy, R Howell, et al. Comparison of CT- and FDG-PET-defined gross tumor volume in intensity-modulated radiotherapy for head-and-neck cancer. Int J Radiat Oncol Biol Phys 61:1385–92, 2005.

37. A van Baardwijk, BG Baumert, G Bosmans, et al. The current status of FDG-PET in tumour volume definition in radiotherapy treatment planning. Cancer Treat Rev 32:245–60, 2006.

38. C Scarfone, WC Lavely, AJ Cmelak, et al. Prospective feasibility trial of radiotherapy target definition for head and neck cancer using 3-dimensional PET and CT imaging. J Nucl Med 45:543–52, 2004.

39. DL Schwartz, E Ford, J Rajendran, et al. FDG-PET/CT imaging for preradiotherapy staging of head-and-neck squamous cell carcinoma. Int J Radiat Oncol Biol Phys 61:129–36, 2005.

40. YK Lee, G Cook, MA Flower, et al. Addition of 18F-FDG-PET scans to radiotherapy planning of thoracic lymphoma. Radiother Oncol 73:277–83, 2004.

41. M Hutchings, A Loft, M Hansen, et al. Clinical impact of FDG-PET/CT in the planning of radiotherapy for early-stage Hodgkin lymphoma. Eur J Haematol 78:206–12, 2007.

42. EV Dizendorf, BG Baumert, GK von Schulthess, et al. Impact of whole-body 18F-FDG PET on staging and managing patients for radiation therapy. J Nucl Med 44:24–29, 2003.

43. E Brianzoni, G Rossi, S Ancidei, et al. Radiotherapy planning: PET/CT scanner performances in the definition of gross tumour volume and clinical target volume. Eur J Nucl Med Mol Imaging 32:1392–99, 2005.

44. S Terezakis, M Hunt, C Schmidtlein, et al. 18FDG-PET with CT scan co-registration for radiation treatment planning for lymphoma patients. Int J Radiat Oncol Biol Phys 69: S535–S36, 2007.

45. G Biti, E Cellai, SM Magrini, et al. Second solid tumors and leukemia after treatment for Hodgkin's disease: an analysis of 1121 patients from a single institution. Int J Radiat Oncol Biol Phys 29:25–31, 1994.

46. M Henry-Amar. Second cancer after the treatment for Hodgkin's disease: a report from the International Database on Hodgkin's Disease. Ann Oncol 3 Suppl 4:117–28, 1992.

47. AJ Swerdlow, AJ Douglas, GV Hudson, et al. Risk of second primary cancers after Hodgkin's disease by type of treatment: analysis of 2846 patients in the British National Lymphoma Investigation. BMJ 304:1137–43, 1992.

48. KA Goodman, S Toner, M Hunt, et al. Intensity-modulated radiotherapy for lymphoma involving the mediastinum. Int J Radiat Oncol Biol Phys 62:198–206, 2005.

49. J Yahalom, P Mauch. The involved field is back: issues in delineating the radiation field in Hodgkin's disease. Ann Oncol 13(Suppl 1):79–83, 2002.

50. M Shahidi, N Kamangari, S Ashley, et al. Site of relapse after chemotherapy alone for stage I and II Hodgkin's disease. Radiother Oncol 78:1–5, 2006.

51. T Girinsky, R van der Maazen, L Specht, et al. Involved-node radiotherapy (INRT) in patients with early Hodgkin lymphoma: concepts and guidelines. Radiother Oncol 79:270–77, 2006.

52. T Girinsky, M Ghalibafian, G Bonniaud, et al. Is FDG-PET scan in patients with early stage Hodgkin lymphoma of any value in the implementation of the involved-node radiotherapy concept and dose painting? Radiother Oncol 85:178–86, 2007.

4 Overview of Systemic Management Options for Hodgkin's and Non-Hodgkin's Lymphoma

John W Sweetenham

Introduction

There have been major improvements in the outcome for patients with Hodgkin's lymphomas (HL) and non-Hodgkin's lymphomas (NHLs) in recent years. Many factors have contributed to this improvement in outcome including advances in diagnostic and staging techniques as well as improved supportive care. The major contributor to improved outcome has been the development of systemic treatments with high anti-tumor activity and reduced short- and long-term toxicity. Systemic therapy using combination chemotherapy (with the addition of monoclonal antibodies in certain lymphoma subtypes) is now the primary treatment modality for most patients with HL and NHL, irrespective of the anatomic extent of their disease. The role of radiation therapy has diminished, although it remains an important component of therapy for certain patients with limited-stage disease.

Although combination chemotherapy remains the primary systemic treatment modality for these diseases, new therapeutic options are now being introduced. Monoclonal antibody therapy has resulted in major improvements in outcome for certain patients with B-cell NHLs. The application of immune-based therapies, including idiotypic vaccination and manipulation of the graft versus lymphoma effect in allogeneic stem cell transplantation (SCT), are under active investigation. The explosion of knowledge of the molecular pathogenesis of lymphoma has resulted in the identification of multiple new rational therapeutic targets for therapy, which are now being investigated in phase I and II clinical trials.

Hodgkin's Lymphoma

Advanced Disease

The use of modern combination chemotherapy or combined modality therapy for HL results in cure rates in excess of 90% in some recently published randomized clinical trials, but concerns about long-term toxicity and excess non-relapse mortality in survivors remain. Achieving high cure rates while minimizing the potential for late therapy-related toxicity is the goal of modern treatment of this disease.

Until the early 1990s, treatments developed from the MOPP (mustine, vincristine, procarbazine, prednisone) [1] regimen, ABVD (doxorubicin, bleomycin, vinblastine, dacarbazine) [2], or alternating or hybrid variants of these two regimens had been tested in multiple randomized clinical trials. The Cancer and Leukemia Group B (CALGB) randomized trial of ABVD versus MOPP versus MOPP alternating with ABVD for advanced Hodgkin's disease demonstrated improved response, disease-free and overall survival (OS) rates for ABVD and MOPP/ABVD when compared with MOPP alone [3]. The lower acute toxicity of the ABVD arm in this study led to the adoption of this regimen as the generally recognized "standard" regimen during the 1990s and up to the present time. In the CALGB study, this regimen produced 5-year disease-free and OS rates of 61 and 75%, respectively.

Higher response and survival rates have been reported recently for novel dose-intensive and dose-dense chemotherapy regimens, including Stanford V [4] and BEACOPP (bleomycin, etoposide, doxorubicin, cyclophosphamide, vincristine, procarbazine, prednisone) [5].

Stanford V

Stanford V is one of several, novel, brief regimens, which was developed to reduce the overall duration of chemotherapy, thereby increasing dose intensity, while at the same time reducing the total cumulative doses of drugs thought to be responsible for long-term effects of treatment, including alkylating agents, bleomycin and anthracycline.

Stanford V is a 12-week regimen that alternates myelosuppressive and non-myelosuppressive drugs. Consolidative radiation therapy is given to sites of disease bulk defined as lymph node masses with a diameter of $\geq$5 cm, mediastinal masses $\geq$1/3 of the transthoracic diameter and macroscopic splenic disease.

For the first 142 patients treated with this regimen in the original single institution study from Stanford, the 5-year disease-free and OS rates were 89 and 96%, respectively [4]. Comparable results were reported in a subsequent multicenter phase II study from the Eastern Co-operative Oncology Group (ECOG) [6]. It is noteworthy that results for patients with clinical stage IIB disease with bulk mediastinal involvement were particularly encouraging with this regimen, with 100% of patients remaining disease free, most likely because of the extent of the involved-field radiation therapy (IFRT) used with this regimen. Of the 142 patients, 129 received radiation therapy, most commonly to the mediastinum and neck.

Grade 3 or 4 neutropenia was observed in 82% of patients in the original report, but grade 4 thrombocytopenia was uncommon (5%). Constipation (11%) and grade 3 neuromuscular toxicity (4%) were also reported. No cases of acute leukemia or myelodysplastic syndrome (MDS) were reported. Although not formally assessed in the original report, effects on reproductive function appeared to be relatively mild. All females <40 years of age resumed normal menstruation after completion of therapy. Although male reproductive function was not investigated systematically, all of those tested after completion of treatment had normo- or oligospermia. Azoospermia was not observed. Forty-three pregnancies were observed in the 142 patients (19 conceptions among 13 males and 24 conceptions among 19 females).

Despite these encouraging data, most patients (91%) received IFRT, predominantly to the mediastinum. These patients will, therefore, be at risk from well-documented late toxicities of this approach, including second solid tumors, such as lung and breast cancer and coronary artery disease [7]. Close follow-up of these patients will be required for many years to determine the extent of late toxicity attributable to this regimen.

The Stanford V regimen is now being compared with ABVD in two on-going randomized trials in the USA and Europe. At present, no mature results are available from these studies.

BEACOPP

The BEACOPP regimen has been extensively investigated by the German Hodgkin Lymphoma Study Group (GHSG) in large-scale randomized clinical trials. The original HD9 study from this group compared BEACOPP with COPP/ABVD, and also with a dose-escalated BEACOPP regimen with higher doses of chemotherapy supported with the use of hematopoietic growth factors [5]. A total of 1201 eligible patients with stage IIB–IV disease were entered onto this study, of whom 1195 were evaluable for response and survival. Accrual to the COPP/ABVD arm was discontinued at 260 patients when an interim analysis demonstrated inferior response and survival rates in this arm compared with the other two arms. In the final analysis of this study, the 5-year FFTF and OS rates for the escalated BEACOPP arm were 87 and 91%, respectively. These were significantly higher than those for either COPP/ABVD or standard BEACOPP.

However, the escalated BEACOPP regimen produced high rates of acute toxicity. More than 90% of patients experienced grade 3 or 4 leucopenia, and 70% experienced grade 3 or 4 thrombocytopenia. Grade 3 or 4 infectious events were reported in 22% of patients.

This regimen has significant long-term toxicity. Nine patients treated with escalated BEACOPP subsequently developed secondary acute leukemia or MDS, for an actuarial rate of 2.5% at 5 years. The reported rate of male infertility after this regimen is 100% and in females over 25 years of age, there is also a 100% infertility rate with a high rate of early menopause [7].

The escalated BEACOPP regimen is currently being compared with ABVD in a randomized trial by the EORTC.

The optimal regimen for advanced HL is still unclear, although ABVD is widely acknowledged as the internal standard. The ideal regimen will produce high rates of tumor control with minimal potential for late toxicity. The "trade off" may be some increased short-term toxicity compared with standard chemotherapy regimens. Recent data suggest that ABVD can be delivered in a dose-intensive schedule without the requirement for dose delay or reductions for leucopenia, and without the use of hematopoietic growth factors [8,9]. This approach is likely to be adopted in new clinical trials and may prove more effective than ABVD given in the standard fashion.

In the setting of advanced disease, the contribution of radiation therapy has been evaluated in multiple trials, particularly for patients with bulky disease at presentation. The published evidence suggests that radiation therapy to areas of initial bulk disease does not improve progression-free survival (PFS) or OS when highly active chemotherapy regimens are used [10].

Prognostic Factors and Risk-adapted Therapy

The development of reliable and reproducible prognostic factors for advanced HL offers the potential to minimize therapy in low-risk patients, while maintaining cure rates. The identification of poor risk groups allow the rational development of novel regimens for those patients with less likelihood of cure with current therapies.

The International Prognostic System (IPS) developed by oncologists is the most widely adopted prognostic model in advanced HL [11]. This model is based on over 5000 patients with advanced disease, with 5-year PFS rates ranging from 84% for those with no adverse factors, to 56% for those with four or more adverse factors. When the results for the Stanford V regimen were analyzed according to the IPS, there was a clearly inferior outcome for patients with three or more risk factors compared with those with two or less. Similarly, in the GHSG HD9 study, patients with poor risk disease according to the IPS, who received COPP/ABVD, had a significantly worse outcome compared with those with good risk disease.

By contrast, there was no difference in PFS or OS according to the IPS risk group, for patients who received escalated BEACOPP chemotherapy.

The clinical utility of these factors is, therefore, unclear in the context of modern chemotherapy regimens. Recent studies have evaluated the potential use of functional imaging with ^{18}F-fluorodeoxyglucose-positron emission tomography (FDG-PET) to evaluate early response in HL as a prognostic factor for PFS and OS. Gallamini et al. have reported that the results of PET scanning after two cycles of ABVD in patients with advanced HL are highly predictive of subsequent PFS and OS, independent of the IPS score [12].

Current studies in advanced HL are therefore being designed to assess the role of treatment intensification in patients with positive "early" PET scans to determine whether outcome in this group can be improved by an early change in therapy.

Response-adapted approaches of this type are likely to be assessed in several future clinical trials.

High-dose Therapy and Stem Cell Transplantation

As described above, current chemotherapy and radiotherapy regimens cure a high proportion of patients with advanced HL. Results of conventional-dose salvage therapy for those who relapse after initial chemotherapy or who have refractory disease are poor. Early studies conducted in patients relapsing after treatment with MOPP showed that re-treatment with MOPP produced second complete response (CR) rates of about 50%, with a median remission duration of 21 months [1].

However, the long-term outcome was poor with only 17% of patients alive at 20 years. Similar results were reported from the Milan group, using ABVD with the 8-year OS for relapsed HL patients treated with salvage chemotherapy being 54, 28 and 8% for patients with relapse after 1 year, within 1 year and with induction failure, respectively [2].

In a randomized study from CALGB, patients who relapsed after initial therapy with ABVD, and were re-treated with MOPP, had a 5-year failure-free survival (FFS) rate of 31%, compared with 15% for those receiving MOPP first line and ABVD at relapse [3].

High-dose therapy (HDT) and autologous stem cell transplantation (ASCT) has been investigated in this situation in single-center phase II studies, multicenter registry-based studies and in prospective, randomized clinical trials. Two randomized trials have confirmed the superiority of high-dose therapy and ASCT. In the larger of these two studies, which included 161 patients, freedom from treatment failure (FFTF) at 3-years was significantly improved in the SCT arm (55 vs. 34%, $p = 0.019$), while OS did not differ significantly between treatment arms (71 vs. 65%, $p = 0.331$) [13]. The failure to demonstrate an OS difference is related to the "cross-over" of patients who relapsed on the conventional-dose arm and were salvaged by ASCT. These results have recently been updated, with median follow-up now to 83 months [14]. The 7-year FFTF rate was higher in the SCT arm (32 vs. 49%). No OS difference was observed (56 vs. 57%, respectively, at 7 years).

The results of these studies have established HDT and ASCT as the standard of care for patients with relapsed HL after a prior chemotherapy regimen, such as MOPP or ABVD, irrespective of the duration of the initial remission. However, with the advent of multi-drug dose-dense and dose-intensive chemotherapy regimens for initial treatment of advanced HL, the role of HDT and ASCT for relapsing patients is becoming less certain. The Stanford V and escalated BEACOPP regimens both result in high rates of remission and disease-free survival, even for poor risk patients with advanced HL. In the phase II study from Stanford, 16 patients subsequently relapsed, of whom 11 underwent HDT and ASCT [4]. The freedom from second relapse in the entire group of 16 patients was 69% at 5 years, suggesting that relapsed patients had a high rate of salvage. The ability to "salvage" patients who relapse after the BEACOPP regimen is not yet determined.

Early Stage
Early-stage HL is highly curable. Combined modality therapy is regarded as the standard approach and produces freedom from progression and OS rates in excess of 90% at 10 years for good risk patients, and 85–90% for patients with unfavorable early-stage disease, however defined.

Various cooperative groups have identified prognostic factors for early-stage disease. At least three prognostic models are in use in various parts of North America and Europe, making comparisons between trials difficult. Additionally, there has not been widespread agreement on what represents the "standard of care" for patients with early-stage HL. The use of ABVD for four cycles followed by IFRT is regarded as a standard approach for patients with clinically staged (CS) IA through CS IIB (non-bulky) disease, but this is not based on data from prospective randomized trials.

In view of concerns for late cardiac and pulmonary toxicity, as well as the risk of second malignancies, especially for patients receiving mediastinal and/or axillary radiation, several groups have investigated the use of less chemotherapy cycles and lower radiation doses for these patients. Two recent randomized studies have demonstrated that it may be possible to omit radiation completely in some patients with favorable risk disease.

The GHSG HD10 trial included a four-way randomization allowing comparison of two versus four cycles of ABVD and 20 vs. 30 Gy of involved-field radiation for patients with favorable risk early-stage HL [15]. No difference was observed according to the number of chemotherapy cycles or the radiation dose. Long-term follow up for patients in this study will be essential to ensure that there is no risk of late relapse as a result of lower doses of chemotherapy or radiation, but the early results of this trial suggest that some patients with early-stage disease may be cured with minimal therapy and with a much lower risk of late effects of chemotherapy or radiation.

The National Cancer Institute of Canada HD6 study compared chemotherapy alone with extended field radiation therapy for a group of patients with favorable risk HL and demonstrated equivalent event free and OS in the chemotherapy-only group, most of whom received only four cycles of ABVD [16]. A study from Memorial Sloan Kettering Cancer Center compared six cycles of ABVD with the same chemotherapy plus IFRT in early-stage HL and showed no difference in PFS or OS [17].

Emerging evidence therefore suggests that certain patients with early-stage HL may not require radiation therapy and may be curable with chemotherapy alone. Current trials are investigating the potential value of functional imaging with FDG-PET to determine early response or to assess residual masses at completion of chemotherapy. In several of these studies, patients with negative functional imaging are being randomized between radiation or no further therapy. Results of these studies may help determine whether PET is sufficiently predictive in this context and whether radiation can be safely omitted from therapy in responsive patients.

Other Systemic Treatment Modalities for Hodgkin's Lymphoma
Monoclonal Antibodies
The chimeric anti-CD20 monoclonal antibody, rituximab, has been investigated in several recent studies of patients with HL. There is a clear rationale for its use in lymphocyte/histiocyte predominant HL, in which the L&H cells are known to be CD20 positive. In classical HL, the rationale for its use has been 2-fold. Firstly, approximately 20–30% of Hodgkin Reed Sternberg (HRS) cells express CD20, making this a rational choice for targeted therapy. Secondly, the background cellular infiltrate in HL comprises many cell types, including CD20-positive B cells. Since there is increasing evidence that the growth and survival of HRS cells is dependent upon survival signals from surrounding B cells, the depletion of these cells using rituximab may result in anti-tumor activity. Early results from phase II studies have demonstrated a response rate of around 30% for patients with relapsed classical HL receiving rituximab as a single agent [18]. A phase II study in which rituximab has been added to ABVD for initial treatment of advanced classical HL has recently been reported and phase III studies incorporating rituximab with chemotherapy as a component of first-line therapy are now in progress in the USA and Europe.

The CD30 antigen has also been investigated as a target for monoclonal antibody therapy in classical HL. Although expressed on almost all HRS cells, levels of expression of CD30 are relatively low, and studies of unconjugated monoclonal antibodies directed against CD30 have been disappointing. More recently, antibody/drug conjugates directed at CD30 have been developed. At least one of these, SGN35, has shown encouraging activity in patients with relapsed/refractory HL and is being evaluated in phase II studies [19].

Targeted Therapies
Molecular studies have identified multiple signaling pathways in HRS cells that are potential targets for therapy. Studies of some of these new targeted agents are now in progress and early-phase studies have demonstrated clinical activity.

Agents targeting various molecules on the NFκB pathway have been evaluated, including bortezomib and several inhibitors of histone deacetylase. Response rates in the 20–30% range have been reported for these agents. The RANK and TRAIL pathways are also being explored. Recent data implicating bcl-2 as an important adverse prognostic factor in HL have led to studies of agents targeted at bcl-2 family members.

Non-Hodgkin's Lymphomas
The current version of the World Health Organization (WHO) classification of NHL recognizes between 30 and 40 separate clinicopathologic entities, with distinct characteristics and for many, specific treatment approaches. Discussion of each NHL subtype is beyond the scope of this chapter, in which follicular lymphoma (FL) and diffuse large B-cell lymphoma (DLBCL) have been chosen as "model" entities to discuss systemic options for indolent and aggressive NHLs, respectively.

Diffuse Large B-cell Lymphoma
Early Stage. Early studies of the treatment of limited-stage DLBCL used involved IFRT, with most patients relapsing at sites distant from the irradiated area. Combination chemotherapy was therefore introduced in addition to radiation therapy in an attempt to control clinically undetected disease at distant sites. The use of combined modality therapy with three cycles of CHOP (cyclophosphamide, doxorubicin, vincristine, prednisone) followed by IFRT was compared with standard chemotherapy using eight cycles of CHOP, in a study from the Southwest Oncology Group (SWOG) [20]. Localized disease was defined as non-bulky stage I or II disease. The 5-year PFS was 77% for the combined modality arm versus 64% for chemotherapy alone ($p = 0.03$). The corresponding figures for OS were 82 and 72% ($p = 0.02$). This study established combined modality therapy with three cycles of CHOP chemotherapy followed by IFRT as the standard of care for most patients with localized DLBCL. However, longer term follow-up of this study has shown that the early survival advantage associated with combined modality therapy has not been maintained.

A recent study from the Groupe d'Etude des Lymphomes de l'Adulte (GELA) included 647 patients with localized aggressive NHL DLBCL, randomized to receive either three cycles of CHOP chemotherapy followed by IFRT or ACVBP (doxorubicin, cyclophosphamide, vindesine, bleomycin, prednisone) chemotherapy followed by methotrexate, etoposide, ifosfamide and cytarabine [21]. The 5-year EFS was 82% in the chemotherapy arm, compared with 74% in the combined modality arm ($p = <0.001$). The corresponding figures for OS were 90 and 81% ($p = 0.001$).

Whether chemotherapy alone is adequate therapy for patients with bulky disease (however defined) is unclear. In a study from ECOG [22], 352 patients with clinical stage I or II disease (including bulky disease) were initially treated with eight cycles of CHOP chemotherapy. Subsequently, patients in complete remission were then randomized to 30 Gy of IFRT or no further therapy. Patients in PR after chemotherapy received 40 Gy of involved-field radiation. The 6-year disease-free survival was 73% for the radiation therapy arm compared with 56% for the observation arm ($p = 0.05$). No OS difference was observed.

Since patients with limited-stage disease represent a heterogeneous patient group, a stage adjusted IPI has recently been proposed to facilitate risk stratification in future studies in early-stage disease. Patients with no adverse risk factors have a projected 5-year OS of approximately 95% when treated with brief duration

chemotherapy (CHOP × 3) and IFRT. Such combined modality therapy should be regarded as the standard approach for this patient group.

By contrast, patients with one adverse factor have a projected 5-year OS rate of around 70% and only 50–60% of those with three or four adverse factors survive for 5 years. Several studies in advanced DLBCL have now demonstrated improvements in disease-free and OS rates by the addition of rituximab to combination chemotherapy such as CHOP. No randomized studies have been reported to date in limited-stage disease. A recent phase II study from SWOG has tested the addition of rituximab to three cycles of CHOP chemotherapy plus IFRT for diffuse aggressive B-cell NHL [23]. The 2- and 4-year PFS rates were 93 and 88%, respectively, with the corresponding OS rates being 95 and 92%. These results compared favorably with an historical series of patients treated with CHOP × 3 plus IFRT using identical selection criteria. Randomized studies will be required to prospectively evaluate the benefit of the addition of rituximab to chemotherapy in this population.

Advanced Stage. Until recently, CHOP was the standard first-line therapy for all patients with DLBCL, mainly on the basis of the SWOG randomized trial, which compared this regimen with three more intensive regimens, showing no difference in response rates, PFS or OS, but a higher toxicity rate in the regimens other than CHOP [24].

In recent years, two novel approaches have been investigated to attempt to improve outcome in patients with advanced stage disease:

• *Dose intensified and dose dense therapy:*
Studies from the German non-Hodgkin's Lymphoma Study Group [25,26] have investigated intensification of the CHOP regimen, either by reducing the treatment duration from 21 to 14 days, or by the addition of etoposide to the standard regimen. The comparison of CHOP21 with CHOP14 and CHOP with the same regimen plus etoposide (CHOEP) was performed using a 2 × 2 factorial design. Separate trials were performed in older and younger patients, using the same study design. The trial in older patients included 689 patients. CHOP14 was shown to be superior to CHOP21 (5-year EFS for CHOP21 was 33 vs. 44% for CHOP14 ($p = 0.003$)). The corresponding rates for OS were 41 vs. 53% ($p = <0.001$). The addition of etoposide had no effect. The corresponding study in 710 younger patients showed no event free or OS benefit for CHOP14 compared with CHOP21, although an EFS benefit was seen for patients receiving CHOP14 compared with those receiving CHOP21. No OS benefit was observed.

• *Consolidative high-dose therapy and autologous stem cell transplantation*
The effectiveness of ASCT as a salvage treatment in aggressive NHL has encouraged many studies of the use of ASCT as a component of first-line therapy, particularly for patients identified as having "poor risk" disease. Many trials are now published, some of these studies are retrospective, subset analyses of clinical trials, which were not initially stratified according to risk groups and not statistically powered to detect differences in subgroup analysis.

Many prospective trials have subsequently been performed, with variable results. Most studies have failed to show an advantage for high-dose consolidation.

In view of the conflicting results that have been reported in studies of first remission transplantation in aggressive NHL, a meta-analysis has recently been conducted [27]. Data from 2018 patients from 13 randomized trials who were evaluable for outcome were available. A significantly higher CR rate was reported for HDT and ASCT, but no differences in EFS or OS were observed. No difference in outcome was seen according to risk group.

Based on these results, HDT and ASCT is not considered a component of first-line therapy in patients with diffuse aggressive lymphoma (including DLBCL), irrespective of risk group.

• *Addition of rituximab to chemotherapy*

The benefit of adding rituximab to CHOP chemotherapy for DLBCL was initially demonstrated in a randomized trial from the GELA [28] in 399 patients aged between 60 and 80 years with DLBCL, who were randomized to receive eight cycles of CHOP chemotherapy, or the same chemotherapy plus rituximab given on Day 1 of each 21-day cycle. The R-CHOP arm was superior to CHOP in terms of CR rate (76 vs. 63%, $p = 0.005$), 2-year EFS (61 vs. 43%, $p = 0.002$) and 2-year OS (70 vs. 57%, $p = 0.007$). The survival advantage for R-CHOP in this trial was observed in all IPI risk groups.

The addition of rituximab to CHOP in elderly patients with DLBCL has also been investigated in an intergroup study in the USA, in which 632 patients aged over 60 years with DLBCL [29] were randomized to six to eight cycles of CHOP, or the same chemotherapy plus rituximab. A second randomization was included for responding patients between observation only, and maintenance rituximab, given once per week for 4 weeks at 6-month intervals for a total of 2 years. There was a significant improvement in 3-year FFS in the R-CHOP arm compared with CHOP (53 vs. 46%, $p = 0.04$) and in the maintenance rituximab arm compared with observation alone. The advantage of maintenance rituximab appeared to be limited to patients who did not receive this agent as part of their induction regimen. No OS differences were observed on the study.

Further evidence for the benefit of the addition of rituximab to chemotherapy has been reported from a retrospective, population-based study from British Columbia, Canada, which has demonstrated higher event free and OS rates for patients with DLBCL since the introduction of rituximab [30]. A benefit for rituximab in younger, low-risk patients has also been shown in the MInT (MabThera International Trial) [31] in Europe.

Further studies will be required to determine whether biological markers, such as bcl-2 protein expression, will reliably predict those patients likely to benefit from the addition of rituximab to chemotherapy.

High-dose Therapy and Autologous Stem Cell Transplantation

The use of HDT and ASCT has been regarded as the standard of care for patients with relapsed DLBCL for over a decade, based on the results of the PARMA randomized trial [32]. This study included 215 patients with relapsed aggressive NHL (mostly DLBCL), initially treated with two cycles of salvage chemotherapy with DHAP (dexamethasone, high-dose cytosine arabinoside, cisplatin).

Responding patients were randomized to receive further DHAP chemotherapy, or to proceed to HDT using BEAC (carmustine, etoposide, cytarabine, cyclophosphamide) and autologous bone marrow transplantation. Significantly superior 5-year event free (46 vs. 12%, $p = 0.0001$) and OS (53 vs. 32%, $p = 0.038$) rates were observed for the transplant arm compared with the conventional chemotherapy arm. The relevance of this study in the present context is unclear. Improved supportive care, including the use of peripheral blood progenitor cells, has reduced the morbidity associated with HDT and extended its use to older patient groups, typically up to 70 or 75 years old. Most centers will now offer ASCT to patients who achieved partial remission (PR) to prior therapy, unlike the PARMA study, in which a previous complete remission was required. Patients now routinely treated with ASCT are therefore more heterogeneous than those in the PARMA study, raising questions concerning the current relevance of this trial. The addition of rituximab to combination chemotherapy regimens, and the advent of accelerated 14-day regimens for first-line treatment have improved disease free and OS in DLBCL. It is not clear whether patients who relapse after these regimens will have the same salvage rates as those treated without monoclonal antibodies.

High-dose therapy and ASCT remains the standard of care for patients with relapsed DLBCL, which is still sensitive to second-line chemotherapy, but the benefit of this approach is unclear and requires re-evaluation.

Allogeneic Stem Cell Transplantation in Diffuse Large B-cell Lymphomas

Only limited data exist regarding the use of allogeneic SCT in aggressive lymphoma, using myeloablative or non-myeloablative conditioning regimens. Comparative studies of allogeneic SCT and ASCT in aggressive NHL have not shown a survival advantage for allogeneic SCT, despite the lower relapse rate in allogeneic patients. In the absence of clear evidence of a clinically relevant graft-versus-lymphoma effect in aggressive NHL, the use of allogeneic SCT should be restricted to research protocols.

Allogeneic transplantation for patients who relapse after autologous transplantation is increasing in use, although there are few data to confirm its benefit. A recent retrospective study from the International Bone Marrow Transplant Registry analyzed results for 114 patients with various subtypes of NHL who received allogeneic SCT after relapse following ASCT, suggesting that the curative potential for this approach is low and that its use should be restricted to patients in prospective trials.

Follicular Lymphoma

For the majority of patients with FL, who present with advanced-stage disease, management has been directed at maintaining patients symptom free and with good quality of life for as long as possible. Until recently, there was no evidence to suggest that available therapies had improved survival in patients with FL. Several recent studies have suggested, however, that the survival for patients with FL is improving, and that this may, in part, be related to the introduction of monoclonal antibody-based therapies [33–35]. In view of these data, there has been a recent trend toward the earlier use of more intensive treatment approaches, although this has yet to be shown to improve survival in prospective studies. The adoption of a 'watch and wait' strategy for asymptomatic, advanced-stage patients with no evidence of organ compromise has been compared with early therapy in three prospective randomized trials, all of which show that there is no survival advantage for early chemotherapy compared with a watch and wait approach in this population [36–38].

Chemotherapy

Single alkylating agent therapy with cyclophosphamide or chlorambucil produces response rates of around 80% in advanced FL, although CRs are rare. Early attempts to improve survival rates with the use of combination chemotherapy showed no survival benefit. The early use of anthracycline-based regimens, such as CHOP, has produced higher overall response rates, but CR rates have typically been similar to those seen with single alkylating agents, and time to progression and OS rates have been equivalent [39].

The use of fludarabine-based initial therapy is also associated with higher clinical and molecular response rates, but no survival advantage has been demonstrated and fludarabine-based therapy is associated with a relatively high risk of opportunistic infection [40]. The bone marrow toxicity of fludarabine can be prolonged and subsequent hematopoietic progenitor cell mobilization can be problematic in patients previously treated with this and other purine analogs.

Chemo-immunotherapy

The addition of rituximab to initial chemotherapy for FL has produced marked improvements in long-term disease-free survival, and in some cases, overall survival. A large randomized trial conducted in Europe compared CVP (cyclophosphamide, vincristine, prednisone) with and without rituximab in patients with previously untreated advanced FL. The overall response rate was significantly higher in the rituximab-containing arm (81 vs. 57%), as was the CR rate (41 vs. 10%). In a recent update of the original study, an OS advantage has been shown for patients receiving rituximab. Other studies, using different induction chemotherapy regimens, have confirmed that the addition of rituximab for first-line therapy improves response rates and OS [4,42].

Maintenance Therapy

Several studies have explored the use of maintenance therapy for patients in first remission after various induction regimens. To date, most available data are for rituximab and interferon. Current studies are exploring the potential use of newer agents such as lenalidomide in this context, but results from these studies are not yet available.

Rituximab

A prospective randomized study from ECOG has demonstrated a PFS and OS benefit for the use of rituximab maintenance in patients who received CVP as remission induction therapy [43]. To date, a similar benefit has not been shown in patients who received rituximab as part of their first-line therapy. Further studies are in progress that will help to clarify the role of maintenance rituximab in patients who received this as a component of first-line therapy.

Preliminary data show that the use of maintenance rituximab after induction with single-agent rituximab is associated with a continued response, such that patients who initially achieve a PR after rituximab can convert to CRs with maintenance therapy. There is no evidence of a survival benefit to this approach. A small randomized study, which compared maintenance rituxan with the use of the same agent at the time of documented disease progression, showed no difference in survival or in the time until the use of another agent in either arm [44]. This is now being assessed in a larger randomized trial by ECOG.

Interferon

The role of interferon maintenance therapy after induction chemotherapy in FL has been the subject of multiple randomized trials and one meta-analysis [45]. Improved OS was associated with the use of interferon maintenance after relatively intensive induction chemotherapy regimens, although these studies were all conducted prior to the introduction of rituximab and their relevance to current therapy is therefore unclear.

Idiotypic Vaccination

The potential to delay recurrence of FL by the use of patient-specific idiotypic vaccines after induction therapy has been studies by several groups, and has recently been evaluated in randomized trials that, so far, have failed to show a survival advantage for this approach.

High-dose Therapy and Autologous Stem Cell Transplantation

Randomized studies of first remission ASCT for FL were mostly conducted prior to the introduction of rituximab into first-line therapy, and their relevance is therefore unclear. The completed studies have shown prolongation of EFS by the use of "early" ASCT, but this has not been reflected in an improvement in OS, partly because of an excess of treatment-related deaths in the transplant arm, particularly from MDS/AML [46,47].

Radio-immunotherapy

In view of the activity of anti-CD20-directed radio-immunotherapy in relapsed FL (see below), it has also been evaluated in the first-line setting. Kaminski et al. reported results of a phase II study of ^{131}I-tositumomab in patients with advanced, previously untreated FL, reporting a high overall response rate of 95%, a CR rate of 75% and a median PFS of over 6 years [48]. Although impressive, these results must be interpreted cautiously since the patient group was very favorable with respect to prognostic factors, and many patients did not meet standard criteria for "requiring" treatment. The use of ^{131}I-tositumomab as consolidation therapy for patients receiving CHOP for advanced FL was evaluated in a SWOG study with encouraging results [49]. This approach is now being compared with CHOP-rituximab in a randomized trial.

Relapsed Follicular Lymphoma

Most treatment modalities that are active in first-line therapy of FL are also active in the relapsed setting. Most patients with FL are likely to receive several different regimens during the course of their disease. Current evidence does not demonstrate an optimal sequence of therapies.

Radio-immunotherapy with ^{131}I-tositumomab and ^{90}Y-ibritumomab tiuxetan has shown activity in this context, but, as yet, these agents have not been shown to improve OS.

High-dose therapy and ASCT is frequently used for patients with relapsed FL and has been the subject of multiple single-center and registry-based reports and a single, small, prospective randomized trial [50]. The randomized trial demonstrated a survival advantage for patients receiving ASCT, but was conducted prior to the introduction of rituximab. Long-term results from two major centers have demonstrated very prolonged DFS and OS in patients with FL receiving HDT and ASCT at first relapse/second remission [51].

Allogeneic SCT has also been evaluated in this setting using both ablative and non-ablative conditioning regimens, but remains an experimental approach.

Novel Systemic Approaches for Lymphoma
The identification of rationale therapeutic targets in lymphoma has resulted in the development of multiple new systemic agents for these diseases in recent years, many of which are now under investigation in phase I and II trials. Their future role is unclear, although it is likely that many of these will gain use either as single agents, added to standard chemo-immunotherapy regimens or as rational combinations used to target multiple converging pathways or to provide multiple "hits" on single pathways. Examples of novel targeted agents under investigation in lymphoma include bortezomib, histone deacetylase inhibitors, agents directed at components of the apoptotic mechanism including XIAP inhibitors and BH3 mimetics, and agents targeting mitotic mechanisms including Aurora kinase inhibitors.

Novel monoclonal antibodies are also under investigation. Some of these represent modifications of existing anti-CD20 monoclonal antibodies, which have a greater ability to recruit host immune responses. Some are directed at novel targets, such as CD80, or include novel conjugates, such as drugs or toxins.

REFERENCES

1. DL Longo, PL Duffey, RC Young, et al. Conventional-dose salvage combination chemotherapy in patients relapsing with Hodgkin's disease after combination chemotherapy: the low probability of cure. J Clin Oncol 10:210–18, 1992.
2. V Bonfante, A Santoro, S Viviani, et al. Outcome of patients with Hodgkin's disease failing MOPP-ABVD. J Clin Oncol 15:528–34, 1997.
3. GP Canellos, JR Anderson, KJ Propert, et al. Chemotherapy of advanced Hodgkin's disease with MOPP, ABVD or MOPP alternating with ABVD. New J Engl Med 327:1478–84, 1992.
4. SJ Horning, RT Hoppe, S Breslin, et al. V Stanford and radiotherapy for locally extensive and advanced Hodgkin's disease: mature results of a prospective clinical trial. J Clin Oncol 20:630–37, 2002.
5. V Diehl, J Franklin, M Pfreundschuh, et al. Standard and increased-dose BEACOPP chemotherapy compared with COPP-ABVD for advanced Hodgkin's disease. New J Engl Med 348:2386–95, 2003.
6. SJ Horning, J Williams, NL Bartlett, et al. Assessment of the V Stanford regimen and consolidative radiotherapy for bulky and advanced Hodgkin's disease: Eastern Co-operative Oncology Group pilot study E1492. J Clin Oncol 18:972–80, 2000.
7. M Sieniawski, T Reineke, A Josting, et al. Assessment of male fertility in patients with Hodgkin's lymphoma treated in the German Hodgkin Study Group (GHSG) clinical trials. Ann Oncol. 2008 Jun 17. [Epub ahead of print].
8. E Boleti, GM Mead. ABVD for Hodgkin's lymphoma: full dose chemotherapy without dose reductions or growth factors. Ann Oncol 18:376–80, 2007.
9. AM Evens, T Ortiz, M Gounder, et al. G-CSF is not necessary to maintain over 99% dose intensity with ABVD in the treatment of Hodgkin lymphoma: low toxicity and excellent outcomes in a 10 year analysis. J Br Haematol 137:545–52, 2007.
10. V Diehl, P Schiller, A Engert, et al. Results of the third interim analysis of the HD12 trial of the GHSG: 8 courses of escalated BEACOPP versus 4 courses of escalated BEACOPP and 4 baseline courses of BEACOPP with or without additive radiotherapy for advanced stage Hodgkin's lymphoma. Blood 102:27a, 2003.
11. D Hasenclever, V Diehl. A prognostic score for advanced Hodgkin's disease. International Prognostic Factors Project on Advanced Hodgkin's Disease. New J Engl Med 339: 1506–14, 1998.
12. A Gallamini, M Hutchings, L Rigacci, et al. Early interim 2-[18F]fluoro-2-deoxy-D-glucose positron emission tomography is prognostically superior to international prognostic score in advanced-stage Hodgkin's lymphoma: a report from a joint Italian-Danish study. J Clin Oncol 25:3746–52, 2007.
13. N Schmitz, B Pfistner, M Sextro, et al. Aggressive conventional chemotherapy compared with high-dose chemotherapy with autologous haemopoietic stem-cell transplantation for relapsed chemosensitive Hodgkin's disease: a randomized trial. Lancet 359:2065–71, 2002.
14. N Schmitz, H Haverkamp, A Josting, et al. Long term follow up in relapsed Hodgkin's disease (HD): updated results of the HD-R1 study comparing conventional chemotherapy (cCT) to high-dose chemotherapy (HDCT) with autologous haemopoietic stem cell transplantation (ASCT) of the German Hodgkin's Study Group (GHSG) and the Working Party Lymphoma of the European Group for Blood and Marrow Transplantation (EBMT). J Clin Oncol 23:562s (abstract), 2005.
15. V Diehl. Hodgkin's disease—from pathology specimen to cure. N J Engl Med. 357:1968–71, 2007.
16. RM Meyer, MK Gospodarowicz, JM Connors, et al. Randomized comparison of ABVD chemotherapy with a strategy that includes radiation therapy in patients with limited-stage Hodgkin's lymphoma: National Cancer Institute of Canada Clinical Trials Group and the Eastern Cooperative Oncology Group. J Clin Oncol 23:4634–42, 2005.
17. DJ Straus, CS Portlock, J Qin, et al. Results of a prospective randomized clinical trial of doxorubicin, bleomycin, vinblastine, and dacarbazine (ABVD) followed by radiation therapy (RT) versus ABVD alone for stages I, II, and IIIA nonbulky Hodgkin disease. Blood 104:3483–89, 2004.
18. A Younes, J Romaguera, F Hagemeister, et al. A pilot study of rituximab in patients with recurrent classic Hodgkin disease. Cancer 98:310–14, 2003.
19. A Younes, A Forero-Torres, NL Bartlett, et al. Objective responses in a phase I dose-escalation study of SGN-35, a novel antibody-drug conjugate (ADC) targeting CD30 in

patients with relapsed or refractory Hodgkin lymphoma. J Clin Oncol 26:460s, 2008.

20. TP Miller, S Dahlberg, JR Cassady, et al. Chemotherapy alone compared to chemotherapy plus radiotherapy for localized intermediate- and high-grade non-Hodgkin's lymphoma. New Engl J Med 339:21–26, 1998.

21. F Reyes, E Lepage, G Ganem, et al. ACVBP versus VHOP plus radiotherapy for localized aggressive lymphoma. New Engl J Med 352:1197–205, 2005.

22. SJ Horning, E Weller, K Kim, et al. Chemotherapy with or without radiotherapy in limited-stage diffuse aggressive non-Hodgkin's lymphoma: Eastern Cooperative Oncology Group Study 1484. J Clin Oncol 22:3032–38, 2004.

23. DO Persky, JM Unger, CM Spier, et al. II Phase study of rituximab plus three cycles of CHOP and involved-field radiotherapy for patients with limited-stage aggressive B-cell lymphoma: Southwest Oncology Group study 0014. J Clin Oncol 26:2258–63, 2008.

24. RI Fisher, ER Gaynor, S Dahlberg, et al. Comparison of a standard regimen (CHOP) with three intensive chemotherapy regimens for advanced non-Hodgkin's lymphoma. New Engl J Med 328:1002–6, 1993.

25. M Pfreundschuh, L Trumper, M Kloess, et al. Two-weekly or 3-weekly CHOP chemotherapy with or without etoposide for the treatment of young patients with good-prognosis (normal LDH) aggressive lymphomas: results of the NHL-B1 trial of the DSHNHL. Blood 104:626–33, 2004.

26. M Preundschuh, L Trumper, M Kloess, et al. Two-weekly or 3-weekly CHOP chemotherapy with or without etoposide for the treatment of elderly patients with aggressive lymphomas: results of the NHL-B2 trial of the DSHNHL. Blood104:634–41, 2004.

27. A Greb, DH Schiefer, J Bohlius, et al. High-dose chemotherapy with autologous stem cell support is not superior to conventional-dose chemotherapy in the first-line treatment of aggressive non-Hodgkin's lymphoma – Results of a comprehensive meta-analysis. Blood 104:263a (abstract), 2004.

28. B Coiffier, E Lepage, J Briere, et al. CHOP chemotherapy plus rituximab compared with CHOP alone in elderly patients with diffuse large B-cell lymphoma. N Engl J Med 346:235–42, 2002.

29. TM Habermann, EA Weller, VA Morrison, et al. Rituximab-CHOP versus CHOP alone or with maintenance rituximab in older patients with diffuse large B-cell lymphoma. J Clin Oncol 24:3121–27, 2006.

30. LH Sehn, J Donaldson, M Chhanabhai, et al. Introduction of combined CHOP plus rituximab therapy dramatically improved outcome of diffuse large B-cell lymphoma In British Columbia. J Clin Oncol 23:5027–33, 2005.

31. M Pfreundschuh, L Trumper, D Gill, et al. First analysis of the completed MabThera International (MInT) trial in young patients with low-risk diffuse large B-cell lymphoma (DLBCL): addition of rituximab to a CHOP-like regimen significantly improves outcome of all patients with the identification of a very favorable subgroup with IPI = 0 and no bulky disease. Blood 104:48a [abstract], 2004.

32. T Philip, C Guglielmi, A Hagenbeek, et al. Autologous bone marrow transplantation as compared with salvage chemotherapy in relapses of chemotherapy-sensitive non-Hodgkin's lymphoma. N Engl J Med. 333:1540–45, 1995.

33. WT Swenson, JE Wooldridge, CF Lynch, et al. Improved survival of follicular lymphoma patients in the United States. J Clin Oncol 23:5019–26, 2005.

34. Q Liu, L Fayad, F Cabanillas, et al. Improvement in overall and failure-free survival in stage IV follicular lymphoma: 25 years of treatment experience at the University of MD Texas Anderson Cancer Center. J Clin Oncol 24:1582–89, 2006.

35. RI Fisher, M LeBlanc, OW Press, et al. New treatment options have changed the survival of patients with follicular lymphoma. J Clin Oncol 23:8447–52, 2005.

36. RC Young, DL Longo, E Glatstein, et al. The treatment of indolent lymphomas: watchful waiting v aggressive combined modality treatment. Semin Hematol 25:11–16, 1988.

37. P Brice, Y Bastion, E Lepage, et al. Comparison in low-tumor-burden follicular lymphomas between an initial no-treatment policy, prednimustine, or interferon alfa: a randomized study from the Groupe d'Etude des Lymphomes Folliculaires. Groupe d'Etude des Lymphomes de l'Adulte. J Clin Oncol 15:1110–17, 1997.

38. KM Ardeshna, P Smith, A Norton, et al. Long-term effect of a watch and wait policy versus immediate systemic treatment for asymptomatic advanced stage non-Hodgkin's lymphoma: a randomized controlled trial. Lancet 362:516–22, 2003.

39. E Kimby, M Bjorkholm, G Gahrton, et al. Chlorambucil/prednisone vs CHOP in symptomatic low grade non-Hodgkin's lymphomas: a randomized trial from the Lymphoma Group of Central Sweden. Ann Oncol 5 (Suppl 2):67–71, 1994.

40. A Hagenbeek, H Eghbali, S Monfardini, et al. III Phase intergroup study of fludarabine phosphate compared with cyclophosphamide, vincristine, and prednisone chemotherapy in newly diagnosed patients with stage III and IV low-grade malignant non-Hodgkin's lymphoma. J Clin Oncol 24:1590–96, 2006.

41. R Marcus, K Imrie, A Belch, et al. CVP chemotherapy plus rituximab compared with CVP as first-line treatment for advanced follicular lymphoma. Blood 105:1417–23, 2005.

42. W Hiddemann, M Kneba, M Dreyling, et al. Frontline therapy with rituximab added to the combination of cyclophosphamide, doxorubicin, vincristine and prednisone (CHOP) significantly improves the outcome for patients with advanced stage follicular lymphoma compared with therapy with CHOP alone: results of a prospective study of the German Low Grade Lymphoma Study Group. Blood 106:3725–32, 2005.

43. HS Hochster, E Weller, RD Gascoyne, et al. Maintenance rituximab after CVP results in superior clinical outcome in advanced follicular lymphoma: results of the E1496 phase III trial from the Eastern Cooperative Oncology Group and the Cancer and Leukemia Group B. Blood 106:106a, 2005.

44. JD Hainsworth, S Litchy, D Shaffer, et al. Maximizing therapeutic benefit of rituximab: maintenance therapy versus re-treatment at progression in patients with indolent non-Hodgkin's lymphoma. A randomized phase II trial of the Minnie Pearl Cancer Research Network. J Clin Oncol 23:1088–95, 2005.

45. AZ Rohatiner, WM Gregory, B Peterson, et al. Meta-analysis to evaluate the role of interferon in follicular lymphoma. J Clin Oncol 23:2215–23, 2005.

46. M Ladetto, P Corrandini, S Vallet, et al. High rate of clinical and molecular remissions in follicular lymphoma patients receiving high-dose sequential chemotherapy and autografting at diagnosis: a multicenter, prospective study by the Gruppo Italiano Trapianto Midollo Osseo (GITMO). Blood 100:1559–65, 2002.

47. G Lenz, M Dreyling, E Schiegnitz, et al. German Low-Grade Lymphoma Study Group. Myeloablative radiochemotherapy followed by autologous stem cell transplantation in first remission prolongs progression-free survival in follicular lymphoma – results of a prospective randomized trial of the German Low-Grade Lymphoma Study Group. Blood 104:2667–74, 2004.

48. MS Kaminski, M Tuck, I Estes, et al. ^{131}I-tositumomab therapy as initial treatment for follicular lymphoma. New Engl J Med 352:441–49, 2005.

49. OW Press, JM Unger, RM Braziel, et al. A phase 2 trial of CHOP chemotherapy followed by tositumomab/iodine 131 tositumomab for previously untreated follicular non-Hodgkin's lymphoma: Southwest Oncology Group protocol S9911. Blood 102:1606–12, 2003.

50. HC Schouten, W Qian, S Kvaloy, et al. High-dose therapy improves progression free survival and survival in relapsed follicular non-Hodgkin's lymphoma: results from the randomized CUP European trial. J Clin Oncol 21:3918–27, 2003.

51. AZ Rohatiner, L Nadler, AJ Davies, et al. Myeloablative therapy with autologous bone marrow transplantation for follicular lymphoma at the time of second or subsequent remission: long-term follow-up. J Clin Oncol 25:2554–59 2007.

5 Hodgkin's Lymphoma: Risk and Response-Adjusted Consolidative Treatment Fields

Nidhi Sharma and Roger M Macklis

Introduction

Radiotherapy has long been a mainstay of Hodgkin's lymphoma (HL) management. In 1902, Pusey reported on the successful response of HL treated with high energy therapeutic radiation [1]. Detailed studies describing control rates, dose-response data and patterns of treatment failure after radiotherapy were more fully described in the subsequent papers of early clinical investigators such as Peters, Kaplan and others [2–4]. Of great clinical significance, HL appeared to be one of those radioresponsive malignancies for which generally predictable patterns of physiologic spread allowed the formulation of reproducible and fairly dependable algorithms for predicting long-term control and ultimate cure. The classic management paradigm involved the need to treat all clinically evident sites of disease plus one additional lymphatic group in each adjacent lymphoid chain. This simplistic "known involved sites plus one more in each direction" algorithm essentially allowed lymphoma radiotherapists to make up for the shortcomings and poor sensitivity of the early staging systems and diagnostic techniques. The megavoltage radiation doses necessary for long-term control of this disease were low enough that relatively large regions of adjacent normal tissue could be safely treated without disastrous long-term toxicity. This demonstration of normal tissue "tolerance" to intermediate doses of therapeutic radiation allowed a large "margin" of clinically uninvolved tissue to be safely included within the treatment field, thereby allowing control of even clinically occult areas of "microscopic" residual disease. Radiation dose levels of 36–44 Gy proved adequate to control gross disease and somewhat lower doses (30–40 Gy) became the accepted management strategy for sub-clinical "microscopic" disease. Treatment protocols based on this pattern of spread and dose levels became generally accepted and specialized megavoltage techniques including customized beam blocking, pre-treatment beam simulation methods, and efficient dose delivery filters and targeting processes allowed control of scattered disease deposits in even highly inhomogeneous tissue. Relapse-free control rates on the order of 85% with ultimate disease control rates on the order of 90–95% became the gold standard for comparing therapeutic outcomes and for benchmarking institutional quality for early-stage HL treated with definitive wide-field radiotherapy.

The development of effective chemotherapy regimens in the 1970s and 1980s dramatically altered the preferred long-term therapeutic strategies for both early- and advanced-stage HL. Multi-agent regimens, such as MOPP, ABVD, and similar cytotoxic combinations [12,13] demonstrated the power and relative safety of using a cocktail of cytotoxic agents with different mechanisms of action and normal tissue toxicities. The development of these new systemic regimens added greatly to the range of therapeutic options available for management of this disease. Although initial combined modality protocols were based on attempts to combine nearly full dose external beam radiotherapy with the maximal tolerable doses of chemotherapy, excessive short- and long-term toxicity levels ultimately modified the general vision of how best to combine these powerful but potentially toxic tumor control mechanisms. Several series of preliminary dose-finding comparisons reached publication and, ultimately, randomized treatment comparisons seeking to determine how best to maximize tumor control rates while staying within acceptable normal tissue toxicity thresholds led to the modern era of chemotherapy dominance for HL management. This paradigm assumes that chemotherapy will represent the mainstay of treatment for both early- and advanced-stage HL with consolidative radiotherapy utilized only sparingly and in selected circumstances. Thus, with the exception of certain very specific clinical situations, such as localized nodular lymphocyte predominant HL, definitive wide-field radiotherapy as a sole modality is now rarely used for frontline HL control. The reason for this paradigm shift is based not so much on concern about disease control, which is usually achievable with well-designed radiotherapy fields, but instead on growing evidence for long-term radiotherapy-related complications, including cardiopulmonary toxicity and treatment field second malignancies such as breast cancer. Clinical trials have now shown virtual equivalence of extended-field full-dose radiotherapy and competitive systemic regimens involving four to eight cycles of chemotherapy followed by smaller low-dose involved-field consolidative radiotherapy. For early-stage HL, radiotherapy is now generally applied selectively to bulky or chemorefractory areas of clinical disease. Current clinical trials have largely incorporated this systemic treatment emphasis; thus, clinical trial arms involving radiotherapy questions are usually designed to determine the minimal safe radiation doses and treatment fields necessary to confer adequate local control rates. Table 5.1 summarizes some of the most important data sets buttressing the current HL conceptual paradigms. In essence, it appears that minimal treatment fields used to deliver radiotherapy doses between 20 and 30 Gy may suffice and may help to minimize iatrogenic complications.

State of the Art: Risk- and Response-adapted Treatment

Many authors have addressed the potential for late complications induced by radiotherapy, and have therefore advocated the use of minimal doses or even chemotherapy alone in order to minimize side effects. Bhatia et al. [5] demonstrated that the risk of second solid tumors, especially breast cancer, is extremely high among women who were treated with radiation for childhood HL. Travis et al. [6] also supported the findings of this study. Similarly, Leeuwen et al. [7] showed an increased risk of breast cancer with an increase in radiation dose up to 40 Gy. Salloum et al. [8] demonstrated that radiotherapy was associated with a statistically significant increase in secondary tumors, particularly lung cancer, whereas chemotherapy alone was not associated with any significant increase in such secondary solid tumors. Other investigators, including Aleman et al. [9], Hancock et al. [10] and

Table 5.1 Important Recent Clinical Protocols Defining Management Strategies for Hodgkin's Lymphoma: Early Stage

Trial	Treatment Arms	Outcomes	
		RFS (%)	OS (%)
Favorable groups – early stage			
Milan Group		12-year	12-year
	ABVD×4 STNI 30 Gy	87	96
	ABVD×4 IF (36–40) Gy		
EORTC – GELA H9F		4-year	4-year
	EBVP×6 IF (36 Gy)	87	98
	EBVP×6 IF (20 Gy)	84	98
	EBVP×6 (closed early)	70	98
Unfavorable groups – early stage			
EORTC – GELA H8-U	MOPP×6/ABV IF (36–40 Gy)	89	90
	MOPP×4/ABV IF (36–40 Gy)	92	94
	MOPP×6/ABV STNI (36–40 Gy)	92	92
EORTC – GELA H8-U	ABVD×4 IF 30 Gy	89	95
	ABVD×6 IF 30 Gy	94	96
	BEACOPP×4 IF 30 Gy	91	93
MSKCC stage I, II, IIIa (non-bulky disease)	ABVD×6	81	90
	ABVD×6 IF 36 Gy	86	97

Radiotherapy doses and fields are variable with unclear roles [32].

Ng et al. [11], showed an increased risk of cardiovascular complications for patients receiving thoracic radiotherapy.

Despite the fact that these late complications were often attributed to outdated radiation doses, fields and techniques, some advocates of chemotherapy-alone regimens pushed for the complete removal of radiation treatment in HL patients, particularly for early-stage disease [12,13]. As a stimulating finding, a recent review by Franklin et al. [14] regarding all randomized controlled, illustrated that the risk of second malignancies was quite similar in patients with early-stage HL treated with chemotherapy alone or combined modality therapies.

Facts Reinforcing the Case for Limited Radiotherapy or Chemotherapy Alone for Certain Low-risk Cases

The study conducted by Strauss and coworkers [15] compared the clinical outcomes of patients with HL (stages IA–IIIA) randomized to receive 6ABVD alone versus 6ABVD with radiotherapy (36 Gy IF-RT or EF-RT). There was no significant difference in freedom from progression (FFP) and overall survival (OS) rates in the two groups. Despite the fact that the study was based on a fairly small study population (152 patients) and was thus underpowered to detect a difference of less than 20% between study arms, some authors [13] seized the opportunity to propose that ABVD alone was adequate and appropriate for frontline management for most patients.

On the other hand, Grupo Argentino de Tratamiento de la Leucemia Aguda and Grupo Latinoamericano de Tratamiento de Hemopatias Malignas [16] conducted a study resulting in a substantially higher disease-free survival (DFS) in early HL patients treated with 6CVPP and local-field radiotherapy in comparison to patients treated with chemotherapy alone. Only in a statistically dubious "sub-group analysis" did they find comparable results for both groups.

Another major randomized study conducted by the National Cancer Institute of Canada Clinical Trials Group and the Eastern

Co-op Oncology Group [17] compared chemotherapy alone (four to six cycles of ABVD) with a strategy comprising fairly extensive radiation therapy (sub-total nodal irradiation; STNI) plus chemotherapy in patients with non-bulky early-stage HL. The 5-year FFP rate was significantly higher in patients who received radiotherapy, but OS was comparable between the two groups.

The degree to which higher FFP rates with combination therapy might be expected to influence survival will depend in large part on the duration of follow-up. Sadly, most randomized studies typically have short follow-up periods suggesting that long-term data re-evaluation will be necessary for future studies.

It seems quite likely that limited-field radiotherapy utilizing relatively low doses given in the modern combined modality treatment setting will tend to benefit the majority of patients. Moreover, harmful chemotherapy drug effects can also be minimized by judicious combined modality treatment regimens, as demonstrated by Donaldson et al. [18] and Landman-Parker et al. [19]. It seems clear that neither chemotherapy nor radiotherapy represent an ideal regimen for all patients with HL. But how can we predict which patients require additional intensity of tumor control?

Response-adapted Treatment Regimens

The development of validated algorithms for risk- and response-adapted therapy regimens may provide optimal balance between therapeutic efficacy and toxicity. This sort of response-adjusted algorithm would reduce overall treatment intensity for highly responsive cases. There exist two different concepts underlying this sort of stratagem.

According to the first approach, the treatment intensity of combined modality therapy should be decreased in all groups of patients (as assessed in a randomized study performed by German Hodgkin's study group HD 13). A combination of various cytotoxic compounds is tested at different intensities along with reduced radiation doses and field sites [20].

The second concept (response-adapted treatment) attempts to modify the treatment intensity for each patient by tailoring the intensity of chemotherapy radiation doses to the degree of response observed. This treatment customization requires defining several pre-requisites:

1. Clinical and biological response criteria including:
   a. Complete remission (CR) [17,18,21–23]
   b. Good response (greater than 75%) [19]

2. Timing of evaluation of tumor response and its predictive value; early response (after two to four cycles) versus more sluggish response (greater than four cycles to achieve maximal effect)

3. Reliable methods for evaluation of tumor responses – computed tomography (CT) and positron emission tomography (PET) scans combined with other indices of tumor clearance – blood tests, presence or absence of systemic symptoms, etc. Several recent studies suggest that the response observed on 2-[18F] fluoro-2-deoxyglucose (FDG)-PET after just two cycles of chemotherapy ("the early look" approach) was highly predictive of eventual clinical outcomes [24,25]

Surrogate End Points

The use of functional imaging in assessing response to candidate therapies represents an extremely important area within oncology.

The identification of optimal disease management algorithms is now driven partially by evidence for disease responsiveness and partially by the degree to which one must invest patient and healthcare service time, effort and resources in identifying treatment strategies that will produce optimal outcomes for a specific patient. Note that the idea of "personalized" treatment algorithms appears almost antithetical to the time-honored PHARMA vision of the quest for "blockbuster" drugs, one-size-fits-all curatives with huge population responsiveness characteristics and medical/financial impact. In the case of malignant lymphoma, a wealth of published data are now emerging, demonstrating ubiquitous disease responsiveness to many varieties of therapeutics, but to varying degrees and often unpredictable response duration. An objective, well-validated, non-invasive test process able to winnow down the candidate therapeutics would be a great boon to the oncologic field. We are now compiling fairly compelling datasets consisting of receiver/operator characteristics (ROC) for functional imaging technology used in the management of many different lymphoma histologies. These sorts of data are especially important for lymphoma histologies, where a radiologic PR based on CT imaging may seem to indicate either a complete cytologic response (perhaps with some residual fibrotic "scar" tissue) or, conversely, a partially treated and still quite viable residual tumor deposit at the nidus of the "scar tissue".

A recent multi-disciplinary panel convened by the American Society of Clinical Oncology (ASCO) was charged with evaluating the state of the evidence for the use of functional imaging, such FDG-PET, in the management of patients with many different tumor types [26]. This panel included members from academia, community practice, professional societies, patient advocacy groups, research foundations and third-party payers. Findings were released in July 2007 and have now received fairly wide publication and discussion. The key focus of the panel related to the evaluation and analysis of the grades of evidence adduced for various clinical functional imaging uses and the reliability and strength of recommendations made on the basis of this relatively new technology. An important observation was made fairly early in the deliberations of the panel regarding the relative importance of statistical validity versus clinical management impact for each specific clinical scenario under discussion. Hilden commented on the philosophical divisions between the hard-core statisticians and "ROC graphers" primarily interested in the accuracy and validity of the ROC observed on the specificity curves obtained for the technology, versus the more humanist-oriented "VOI graphers" who believed that the focus of the discussion should instead rest on the evaluation of the potential clinical values and the somewhat subjective impact levels of the decision making, developing overall management strategies for optimal outcomes for specific patients. The relevant data sets included, for each clinical situation, the sensitivity, specificity and likelihood ratio of the evaluated test's ability to successfully predict clinical outcomes. From malignant lymphoma, the great variability of different individual histologies for the FDG-PET sequestration effect makes this topic especially complex. False positives and post-treatment inflammatory responses require that adequate amounts of time elapse between the use of the specific therapeutic modality under evaluation and the subsequent biophysical interrogation using FDG-PET or similar non-invasive testing. For FDG-PET, the optimal interval is often considered to be 4–8 weeks after most recent therapy and

earlier testing may yield confusing false positives. Unfortunately, for the practicing oncologist, waiting 4–8 weeks after a cycle of treatment (either chemotherapy or radiotherapy) may yield substantial neoplastic re-growth; thus, there is a tension between the desire to perform the functional imaging study as soon as feasible after a course of treatment is administered versus the need to wait a sufficient period of time to get a valid report on disease response at the site of interest. An important area of focus for oncologists and healthcare planners is the area of "surrogate clinical endpoints". Clinical oncology funding is often said to require several 100 million dollars per compound for new treatments, which must undergo full clinical testing through phase I, II and III multi-center evaluations. Moreover, the use of validated "early look" test procedures, in which patients are subjected to only a small initial part of a planned multi-month treatment regimen and are then exposed to early-look testing meant to determine whether there is a greater or lesser likelihood that the treatment strategy, if carried to completion, will ultimately result in the desired outcome. Functional imaging tests, such as FDG-PET, are especially interesting in this regard, since these technologies generally measure biochemical and metabolic events that may poorly visualized using more standard anatomic imaging procedures. If functional imaging could be used as a validated "early look" at a time when therapeutic strategies could still be changed, the potential for outcome improvements and a decrease in both toxicity and treatment costs for ultimately futile therapies would be enormous. Moreover, the treatment toxicities and the personal/familial turmoil produced by continuing to press on with futile oncologic endeavors may be responsible for the profound societal fear of cancer when viewed as a disease process. The development of validated non-invasive surrogate endpoints using functional imaging and similar methodologies could dramatically increase the willingness of patient groups, medical advocates and clinical investigators to change course and optimize strategy in an attempt to develop truly "personalized medicine" for effective cancer care, rather than sticking with a prolonged course of ineffective but well-investigated old pharmacologic warhorses.

New Concept Guidelines for Modern Radiotherapy Fields for the Management of Hodgkin's Lymphoma

As discussed earlier in this chapter, both chemotherapy and radiotherapy have the potential for producing unfortunate and, in some cases, irreversible complications, including second cancers. The number of patients with these complications increases as the follow-up period lengthens [27]. Fortunately, it appears that limiting radiation field volume and dose can dramatically reduce the number and severity of many types of treatment complications [14,28–30].

What should Hodgkin's Lymphoma Risk- and Response-adapted Image-guided Radiotherapy Fields look like?

Yahalom and Mauch [31] defined their concept of 'involved fields' though their delineation was not well standardized and was based on Ann Arbor staging. The use of this sort of treatment field demarcation does not fully correlate with our current ability to selectively identify and irradiate specific nodal sites.

A concept thus emerged from the EORTC group planning, namely, involved node radiotherapy (INRT), in which only the initial tumor volume (or involved nodes) receives radiation, thus permitting maximal surrounding normal tissue sparing. This is especially relevant to the desire to limit irradiation of "innocent bystander" structures like heart, lung and breast tissue.

This modern radiotherapy approach involves smaller radiation fields and complex image-guided radiation delivery techniques, when combined with judicious choices for the intensity of chemotherapy, the chance for major improvements in treatment outcomes is clear. The new INRT guidelines [32] will be used in the upcoming EORTC GELA H10 randomized trial.

Basic Rules for Implementing New Guidelines

The following rubric would be relevant for the use of these new "best practice" guidelines:

1. A pre- and post-chemotherapy CT and FDG-PET (generally obtained via an integrated PET-CT platform) should be performed using validated study techniques applied to patients in the treatment position
2. The scans should incorporate cervical, axillary and mediastinal areas
3. All radiologic data should be evaluated by a team including experienced radiologists and nuclear medicine physicians
4. FDG-PET should be used to examine clinically normal-appearing lymph nodes on CT scan images
5. For all initially involved lymph nodes detected on CT or PET scan, the remission status (Cotswold's criteria) after chemotherapy should be identified and compared over time

**Design of Fields Following Complete Response
(or Unconfirmed Complete Response) after Chemotherapy**

An initial clinical target volume (CTV) is first contoured on the radiotherapy planning CT or PET-CT scan. In this model, the CTV is the initial volume of the involved PET positive or grossly enlarged lymph nodes before chemotherapy. Thus the initial pre-chemo PET-CT which will essentially define the CTV takes into account the initial location and extent of all original sites of disease. Normal extranodal structures displaced by enlarged lymph nodes are not typically included in the CTV (e.g., neck muscles). Virtually all PET-positive regions are considered involved or at high risk. Also, whenever possible, large blood vessels and non-involved joints are spared if the involved lymph nodes are located at sufficient distance from them. In case of unconfirmed complete response (Cru), the visible lymph node remnant (scar tissue) is included in the CTV. If a mediastinal area is in CR, the CTV should not exceed the lateral boundaries of the normal mediastinum in order to limit lung toxicity. In other words, the extent of the CTV is essentially defined by the length of the mediastinal mass (or lymph nodes) prior to chemotherapy and the width of the CTV is more similar to the width of the mediastinal mass after chemotherapy. Whenever possible (notably when normal organs are displaced by the initial tumor masses), large thoracic blood vessels, the origins of the coronary arteries and cardiac cavities should not be included in the field. The planning target volume (PTV1) is the CTV with a margin taking into account organ movement and setup variations. A 1-cm isotropic margin is usually considered adequate.

Design of Fields after Partial Response

In this model, the gross tumor volume (GTV) is defined by the lymph node remnant ("scar tissue") after chemotherapy. The CTV is the initial volume before chemotherapy, as described earlier, thereby including the GTV. If a mediastinal area is in partial response (PR), the lateral borders of the irradiated volume will exceed the normal mediastinal boundaries, but its width will be that of the mediastinal mass after chemotherapy. Two PTVs can be defined. PTV1 is the CTV (including the GTV) with a 1-cm isotropic margin. PTV2 is the GTV with a 1-cm isotropic margin, and only PTV2 will ordinarily require an additional radiation boost. (Fig. 5.1a, b).

If initially involved lymph nodes are situated reasonably far apart (more than 5 cm), then separate PTVs are usually

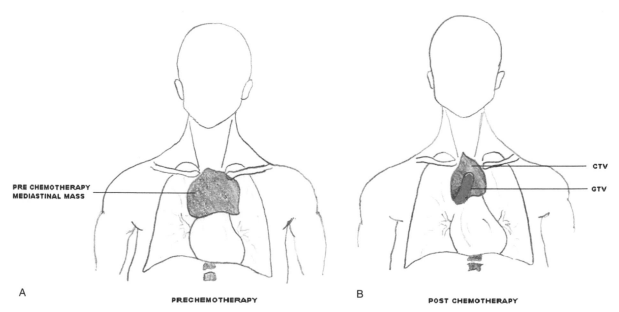

Figure 5.1 (A) The shaded region in the figure depicts the original pre-chemotherapy mediastinal mass as indicated on pre-chemo PET-CT scan. (B) Estimated position of previously involved mediastinal tissue now collapsed into central region after chemotherapy. Shaded region indicates CTV. Residual pseudo-GTV indicated by current position of residual "scar tissue" after chemotherapy. Note that the entire mass is now FDG-negative on PET. Current CCF protocol is to give 2520 cGy to CTV with boost to 3060 cGy for pseudo-GTV region (green shaded region).

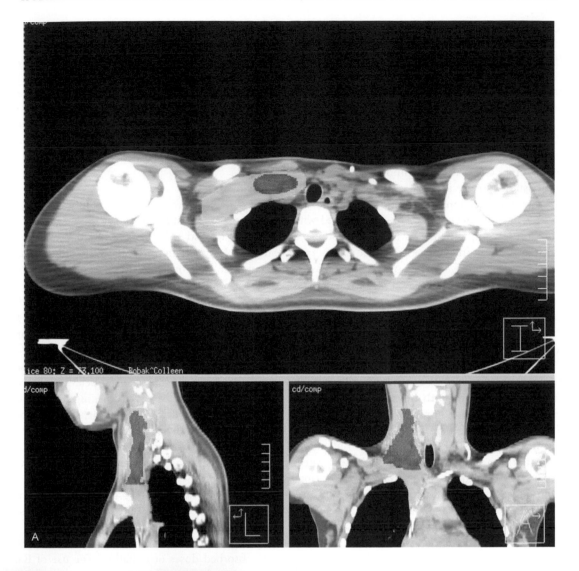

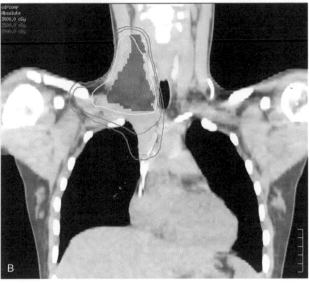

Figure 5.2A, 2B 32 year old woman diagnosed with IIA HL (NS subtype) with PET-CT showing disease in the R neck and supraclavicular regions. The patient had a somewhat sluggish near-CR after 6 cycles of ABVD chemotherapy and post-chemo PET-CT showed no remaining FDG-avid regions. A treatment plan was developed to deliver a dose of approx 2520 cGy to the original PET + regions of adenopathy with a boost to 3060 cGy to the final PET-negative but still somewhat abnormal soft tissue ("scar tissue pseudo-GTV"). Final treatment plan shown in Fig 5.2b (coronal image).

devised; otherwise, they can be included in the same radiation field. According to the International Commission on Radiation Units and Measurements 50/62 [33], the PTV should ordinarily receive a dose comprising between 95 and 107% of the intended prescription dose. The present EORTC-GELA guidelines specify a radiation dose of 30 Gy to PTV1 and an additional 6 Gy radiation boost to PTV2. Other protocols are currently exploring lower doses. At the Cleveland Clinic, we are currently utilizing a dose of 2000–2520 cGy to the initial (PET positive) CTV and a possible boost of an additional 540 cGy to the post-chemotherapy PET-negative GTV (final dose typically 1980 cGy–3060 cGy in 180 or 200 cGy fractions). If some areas remain PET positive after chemotherapy, they may occasionally be boosted to a final dose of 3600 cGy. Fig. 5.2 (a,b) illustrates an example of treatment plan design.

New Radiation Delivery Techniques
Rationale
Smaller fields enable more conformal and innovative approaches to reduce normal tissue exposure and thus should theoretically lower the risk of late complications. This approach could best be implemented by using the new INRT concept coupled with sophisticated radiation techniques, such as intensity-modulated radiation therapy (IMRT) or image-guided radiation therapy (IGRT)-related respiratory gating for HL mediastinal masses. Though not yet fully supported by validated clinical data, this approach should theoretically lower the risk of long-term cardiopulmonary toxicity and/or coronary artery disease. Goodman and coworkers showed that, in such patients, IMRT provided better PTV coverage and reduced pulmonary toxicity (decreased mean dose to lungs by 12–14%) compared with conventional treatments or three-dimensional (3D) conformal radiotherapy. IMRT was also shown to be significantly better in terms of heart and coronary artery protection compared with conventional treatments or 3D-conformal radiotherapy [34].

Two additional features of IMRT/IGRT merit consideration. First, tighter conformal tumor coverage and thus better protection of nearby organs at risk, can often be achieved with various "virtual target volumes" to which selective dose constraints are assigned [35]. The use of serial image datasets can often suggest the kinetics of tumor response to the preliminary chemotherapy, thus helping to differentiate between active tumor and residual inactive "scar tissue". Second, IMRT/IGRT techniques allow radiation oncologists to deliver larger radiation doses to areas considered at a higher risk of local recurrence (risk-adjusted dose painting). These target areas, which are defined by functional imaging using various probes to detect either hypoxic or high proliferation areas, could then be treated with a concurrent boost dose. A note of caution is nevertheless required with IMRT. First, because IMRT produces tighter conformal doses with a steep dose gradient, significant under-coverage of the PTV may occur in patients whose chest organ movements are neither monitored nor controlled. This target motion concern was recently addressed by Duan and coworkers [36]. They showed that IMRT treatments can be affected by respiratory motion, resulting in significant dose errors in individual field doses. However, these errors tend to blur out between fields and local dose inhomogeneity tends to smooth out over a fully fractionated course of treatment. The conclusion was that tumors affected by respiratory motion could be treated with IMRT without clinically significant dosimetric and biological consequences. Very recent results from Girinsky and others relating to treatment of patients with HL and bulky mediastinal masses treated upfront with IMRT (32–40 Gy) after three to six cycles of ABVD suggest that IMRT can be safely administered to such patients despite dosimetric concerns [35]. It is noteworthy that the use of sophisticated radiation delivery techniques may not be devoid of problems because of prolonged radiation delivery times and, thus, lower actual treatment dose rates.

Fowler and coworkers [37] suggested that any prolonged fraction delivery could lead to a possible decrease in the biological effect. Brincker and Bentzen [38], however, showed that sensitivity to changes in the dose per fraction was low in HL. This finding suggests that the capacity to repair sub-lethal damage appears to be small, thus, prolonged radiation delivery should not compromise tumor eradication.

Conclusions
A reasonable view of modern combined modality therapy in the management of HL will incorporate knowledge of the potential benefits and risks of over-reliance on any single cytotoxic strategy. For patients with relatively bulky disease, conventional chemotherapy alone may not produce ideal long-term control rates. However, as therapeutic radiation is potentially toxic, both physiologically and genetically, it must be used sparingly, especially around sensitive normal tissues such as lung and breast. The combination of functional imaging and non-uniform beam delivery techniques will allow risk- and response-adjusted therapy and more personalized approaches to optimal tumor control. The goal is to develop a sort of theoretical "risk matrix" in which the clinician is able to use serial imaging datasets (both volumetric and functional) to decide on whether the likelihood of tumor progression at any individual site is sufficiently high to outweigh the known iatrogenic toxicities of therapeutic radiation. At present, it appears that most experienced lymphoma radiotherapists are incorporating the entire initial area of the disease involvement (suggested on both FDG-PET and on CT evaluations) into an "involved field" or even "involved nodes" version of an initial pre-chemotherapy area at risk, and then using this information to guide the placement of relatively low (approximately 20–30 Gy) absorbed doses of radiation. The use of IGRT/IMRT beam delivery approaches allows further decreases in the dose intensity and volume of irradiated tissue. The current era of risk-adjusted management implies that gradually only the most relapse-prone parts of the original CTV will require more than minimal radiation doses. In some cases, the necessary dose may be zero, but at present the standard of care still calls for at least some consolidative limited field radiotherapy for most cases, especially in an area of initially bulky disease.

REFERENCES
1. WE Pusey. Cases of sarcoma and of Hodgkin's disease treated by exposures to x-rays—a preliminary report. JAMA 38: 166–69, 1902.
2. V Peters. A study of Hodgkin's disease treated radiologically. Am J Roentgenol 63:299–311, 1950.
3. H Kaplan. The radical radiotherapy of Hodgkin's disease. Radiology 78:553–61, 1962.
4. LF Craver. Reflections on malignant lymphoma; Janeway lecture, 1956. Am J Roentgenol Radium Ther Nucl Med 76(5): 849–58, 1956.
5. S Bhatia, LL Robison, O Oberlin. Breast cancer and other second neoplasms after childhood Hodgkin disease. N Engl J Med 334:745–51, 1996.

6. LB Travis, D Hill, GM Dores. Cumulative absolute breast cancer risk for young women treated for Hodgkin lymphoma. J Natl Cancer Inst 97:1428–36, 2005.

7. FE van Leeuwen, WJ Klokman, M Stovall. Role of radiation dose, chemotherapy, and hormonal factors in breast cancer following Hodgkin's disease. J Natl Cancer Inst 95:971–80, 2003.

8. E Salloum, R Doria, W Schubert. Second solid tumors in patients with Hodgkin disease cured after radiation or chemotherapy plus adjuvant low-dose radiation. J Clin Oncol 14: 2435–43, 1996.

9. BMP Aleman, AW van den Belt-Dusebout, WJ Klokman. Long-term cause-specific mortality of patients treated for Hodgkin disease. J Clin Oncol 21:3431–39, 2003.

10. SL Hancock, MA Tucker, RT Hoppe. Factors affecting late mortality from heart disease after treatment of Hodgkin disease. JAMA 270:1949–55, 1993.

11. AK Ng, MP Bernardo, E Weller. Long-term survival and competing causes of death in patients with early-stage Hodgkin disease treated at age 50 or younger. J Clin Oncol 20:2101–8, 2002.

12. DL Longo. Radiation therapy in Hodgkin disease: why risk a pyrrhic victory? J Natl Cancer Inst 97:1394–95, 2005.

13. DL Longo. Hodgkin disease: the sword of Damocles resheathed. Blood 104:3418, 2004.

14. JG Franklin, MD Paus, A Pluctschow. Chemotherapy, radiotherapy and combined modality for Hodgkin disease with emphasis on second cancer risk. The Cochrane Collaboration. Cochrane Library. Eds Wiley; 2006: issue 2.

15. DJ Straus, CS Portlock, J Qin. Results of a prospective randomized clinical trial of doxorubicin, bleomycin, vinblastine, and dacarbazine (ABVD) followed by radiation therapy (RT) versus ABVD alone for stages I, II, and IIIA nonbulky Hodgkin disease. Blood 104:3483–89, 2004.

16. S Pavlovsky, M Maschio, MT Santarelli. Randomized trial of chemotherapy versus chemotherapy plus radiotherapy for stage I–II Hodgkin disease. J Natl Cancer Inst 80:1466–73, 1988.

17. RM Meyer, MK Gospodarowicz, JM Connors. Randomized comparison of ABVD chemotherapy with a strategy that includes radiation therapy in patients with limited-stage Hodgkin lymphoma: National Cancer Institute of Canada Clinical Trials Group and the Eastern Cooperative Oncology Group. J Clin Oncol 23:4634–42, 2005.

18. SS Donaldson, MM Hudson, KR Lamborn. VAMP and low dose, involved-field radiation for children and adolescents with favorable, early-stage Hodgkin disease: results of a prospective clinical trial. J Clin Oncol 20:3081–87, 2002.

19. J Landman-Parker, H Pacquement, T Leblanc. Localized childhood Hodgkin disease: response-adapted chemotherapy with etoposide, bleomycin, vinblastine and prednisone before low-dose radiation therapy: results of the French Society of Pediatric Oncology Study MDH90. J Clin Oncol 18:1500–7, 2000.

20. B Klimm, V Diehl, B Pfistner. Current strategies of the German Hodgkin Study Group (GHSG). Eur J Haematol 75(Suppl 66): 125–34, 2005.

21. FH Kung, CL Schwartz, CR Ferree. POG 8625: a randomized trial comparing chemotherapy with chemoradiotherapy for children and adolescents with stage I, IIA, IIIA1, Hodgkin disease: a report from the Children's Oncology Group. J Pediatr Hematol Oncol 28:362–68, 2006.

22. U Rühl, M Albrecht, K Dieckmann. Response-adapted radiotherapy in the treatment of pediatric Hodgkin disease: an interim report at 5 years of the German GPOH-HD 95 trial. Int J Radiat Oncol Biol Phys 51:1209–18, 2001.

23. MA Weiner, B Leventhal, ML Brecher. Randomized study of intensive MOPP-ABVD with or without low-dose total-nodal irradiation therapy in the treatment of stages IIB, IIIA2, IIIB, and IV Hodgkin disease in pediatric patients: a Pediatric Oncology Group Study. J Clin Oncol 15:2769–79, 1997.

24. M Hutchings, A Loft, M Hansen. FDG-PET after two cycles of chemotherapy predicts treatment failure and progression-free survival in Hodgkin lymphoma. Blood 107:52–59, 2006.

25. A Gallamini, L Rigacci, F Merli. The predictive value of positron emission tomography scanning performed after two courses of standard therapy on treatment outcome in advanced stage Hodgkin disease. Haematologica 91:475–81, 2006.

26. J Gralow, RF Ozols, DF Bajorin et al. Clinical cancer advances 2007: major research advances in cancer treatment, prevention and screening—A report from the American Society of Clinical Oncology. J Clin Oncol 26(8):1394, 2008.

27. NY Mudie, AJ Swerdlow, CD Higgins. Risk of second malignancy after non-Hodgkin lymphoma: a British Cohort Study. J Clin Oncol 24:1568–74, 2006.

28. F Koontz, P Kirkpatrick, W Clough. Combined modality therapy versus radiotherapy alone for treatment of early stage Hodgkin disease: cure versus complications. J Clin Oncol 24: 605–11, 2005.

29. A Engert, P Schiller, A Josting. Involved-field radiotherapy is equally effective and less toxic compared with extended-field radiotherapy after four cycles of chemotherapy in patients with early-stage unfavourable Hodgkin lymphoma: results of the HD8 trial of the German Hodgkin Lymphoma Study Group. J Clin Oncol 21:3601–8, 2003.

30. GM Chronowski, RB Wilder, SL Tucker. Analysis of in-field control and late toxicity for adults with early-stage Hodgkin disease treated with chemotherapy followed by radiotherapy. Int J Radiat Oncol Biol Phys 55:36–43, 2003.

31. J Yahalom, P Mauch. The involved field is back: issues in delineating the radiation field in Hodgkin disease. Ann Oncol 13(Suppl 1):79–83, 2002.

32. T Girinsky, R van der Maazen, L Specht. Involved-node radiotherapy (INRT) in patients with early Hodgkin lymphoma: concepts and guidelines. Radiother Oncol 79:270–77, 2006.

33. ICRU. Prescribing, recording and reporting photon beam therapy. Report 50. Washington, DC: International Commission on Radiation Units and Measurements; 1993.

34. T Girinsky, C Pichenot, A Beaudre. Is intensity-modulated radiotherapy better than conventional radiation treatment and three-conformal radiotherapy for mediastinal masses in patients with Hodgkin disease, and is there a role for beam orientation optimisation and dose constraints assigned to

virtual volumes? Int J Radiat Oncol Biol Phys 64:218–26, 2006.

35. T Girinsky, R van der Maazen, L Specht. Involved-node radio-therapy (INRT) in patients with early Hodgkin lymphoma: concepts and guidelines (author reply). Radiother Oncol 82(1):108–9, 2007.

36. J Duan, S Shen, JB Fiveash. Dosimetric and radiobiological impact of dose fractionation on respiratory motion induced IMRT delivery errors: a volumetric dose measurement study. Med Phys 33:1380–87, 2006.

37. JF Fowler, JS Welsh, SP Howard. Loss of biological effect in prolonged fraction delivery. Int J Radiat Oncol Biol Phys 59:242–49, 2004.

38. H Brincker, SM Bentzen. A re-analysis of available dose-response and time-dose data in Hodgkin disease. Radiother Oncol 30:227–30, 1994.

6 Low Grade and Follicular Histologies
Nidhi Sharma and Roger M Macklis

Introduction

For cases of low-grade B-cell non-Hodgkin's lymphoma (NHL), such as follicular and mucosa-associated lymphoid tissue (MALT) types, up to one quarter of patients will present with early stage (stage 1–2) disease [1]. When appropriately staged, many of these cases will be found appropriate for definitive treatment with local field radiotherapy alone [2]. In recent years, many of the apparently localized cases have been found to harbor occult abnormalities, such as chromosomal changes suggesting systemic involvement, thus implying a high likelihood of disease persistence despite clinically negative initial staging or restaging evaluations [3]. However, even with these molecular indications of occult disease dissemination, many such patients may have a prolonged clinical remission after local therapy alone. It is thus still appropriate to consider definitive local field radiotherapy for early-stage disease as well as symptom-prompted palliative radiotherapy for this clinical group [1–3]. Radiotherapy thus remains an important part of the therapeutic regimens (both focal external beam treatment or, in certain cases, systemic targeted radiopharmaceutical therapy such as radioimmunotherapy; RIT) for patients with localized and more advanced disease stages.

Prognosis and Follicular Lymphoma International Prognostic Index

Prognoses for patients in this disease group are notoriously difficult to predict, but the Follicular Lymphoma International Prognostic Index (FLIPI) gives a reasonable survival estimate [4]. This index, developed in analogy to the better known IPI prognostic system validated for aggressive lymphoma, is based on five adverse prognostic factors [5]. These factors are:

- Number of disease sites (four or more associated with worse prognosis)
- Abnormal LDH (higher worse)
- Patient age (greater than 60 worse)
- The stage (stage 3–4 worse)
- Anemia (hemoglobin less than 12 worse)

The presence of each of these poor prognostic factors confers one risk point; FLIPI score statistics show that patients with a score of 0–1 have expected 10-year overall survivals (OS) in excess of 70%. As one might expect, patients with highly localized disease are often the ones with the low FLIPI score and long expected survivals, thus it makes good sense to offer an attempt at long-term control with highly conformal local field radiotherapy.

Treatment Approaches for Early-stage Indolent non-Hodgkin's Lymphoma

For early-stage disease, focal external beam radiation therapy (XRT) remains a reasonable treatment approach, either with or without the addition of systemic treatments. For radiotherapy alone, multiple published series suggest a 10-year survival probability of approximately 40–50% relapse-free survival (RFS)

and 50–70% OS [5–7]. When systemic therapy is added (either chemotherapy or antibody-based treatment or a combination of the two) significantly higher RFS and OS figures are reported for the group. When only those patients with a higher FLIPI score are considered, systemic therapy, including Rituxan, appears to be substantially more effective than radiotherapy alone. The combination of external beam radiotherapy plus rituximab is currently being investigated both on clinical trials and off-study. Specific information on treatment approaches and outcomes for extranodal B-cell is discussed in the various individual specialized site chapters.

Functional Imaging and Low-grade B-cell non-Hodgkin's Lymphoma

Though ^{18}F-fluorodeoxyglucose-positron emission-tomography (FDG-PET) imaging appears especially useful for higher grade aggressive NHL and Hodgkin's lymphoma (HL), the more indolent NHL subtypes often also demonstrate a moderate or variable degree of FDG avidity [8]. This characteristic FDG sequestration typically occurs at a lower standardized uptake value (SUV) level than that seen in more aggressive varieties of NHL. Because FDG-PET has a reasonably low sensitivity for this disease group, the technology plays a lesser role in the clinical management of low-grade B-cell NHL when compared to the much higher specificity and sensitivity for aggressive NHL and HL.

Radiation Response for Nodal Low-grade B-cell non-Hodgkin's Lymphoma

It has long been appreciated that nodal low-grade B-cell NHL, such as follicular and MALT types, are highly radiosensitive and thus often locally controllable in greater than 90% of cases with clinically localized disease [9]. Doses required for local control are generally on the order of 20–40 Gy. Some of the most reliable data sets, such as those from Stanford University and Princess Margaret Hospital, confirm local control rates of approximately 90% and 10-year RFS rates of up to 50% with overall 10-year survival approaching 75% [10]. Certain groups of patients treated using much lower doses of radiation may also show prolonged clinical disease response. For instance, patients treated for localized follicular NHL receiving just two fractions of 2 Gy each (separated in some cases by several days), may also show gradual disease shrinkage, leading to ultimate regional disease control [11]. This abbreviated course of XRT may be particularly useful for salvage treatment of patients who relapse after full conventional doses of radiotherapy. This approach is especially appealing for patients with adenopathy near some critical normal tissues, such as head and neck. In many cases, this sort of short course, brief re-treatment confers prolonged control while avoiding major toxicity.

Image-guided Radiation Therapy Techniques for Indolent (low-grade) B-cell Nodal non-Hodgkin's Lymphoma

Few published series have dealt specifically with the incorporation of functional imaging techniques, such FDG-PET, into

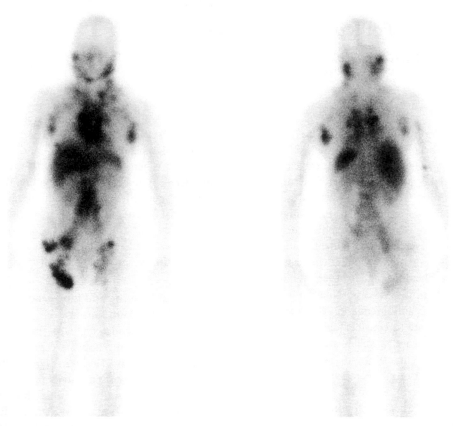

Figure 6.1 Gamma camera image of low grade follicular B cell lymphoma patient imaged using indium-111 ibritumomab ("Zevalin") anti CD20 antibodies in preparation for 90-Y therapeutic Zevalin treatment.

image-guided radiation therapy (IGRT) treatment planning for low-grade nodal NHL patients. This is due in part to the variability of the FDG response in this group and to the copious clinical information using relatively simple anatomic computed tomography (CT) criteria for field design and restaging algorithms. The incorporation of intensity-modulated radiation therapy (IMRT) approaches and the use of strictly limited target volumes

(i.e., limited "involved field" or even the more constrained "involved node") [12] are currently being investigated in many academic sites, but may be unnecessarily complex where doses are low. The use of high precision multi-dimension treatment fields is probably best done on organized clinical trials given the fact that multiple clinically non-enlarged and non-FDG-avid lymph nodes may harbor occult disease and may thus be

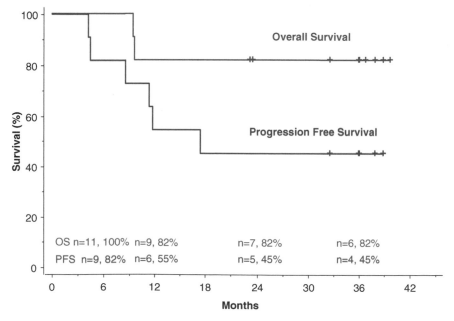

Figure 6.2 Kaplan-Meier progression-free survival (PFS) curve (blue) and overall survival (OS) curve (red) for eleven patients with relapsed or refractory bulky follicular lymphoma treated with external beam radiation therapy followed by yttrium-90 ibritumomab tiuxetan on a Preliminary Phase I-II Clinical Trial.

under-dosed if the treatment field is strictly limited to only those nodes showing clear-cut indication of disease involvement. The general enthusiasm for limiting the size of radiotherapy treatment fields does, however, apply to this patient group as well. As is the case with HL, there is currently intense academic and patient group interest in limiting treatment volumes and in the deliberate use of grossly inhomogeneous radiotherapy field design and "dose painting" meant to match delivered radiotherapy doses with the perceived risk of tumor recurrence and/or serious toxicity at each specific anatomic site [13]. For instance, Ghalilibrifion and colleagues are currently investigating the use of selective IMRT dose delivery plans using radiotherapy fields and normal tissue blocking patterns meant to protect the vascular beds for the coronary arteries in patients undergoing mediastinal radiotherapy [14]. This sort of selective small-field shielding will likely result in a decreased effective dose deposited in certain regions known to be at risk for tumor recurrence, and thus recurrence rates may actually increase. However, on balance, patients and their physicians appear to be in favor of minimizing late radiotherapy toxicity, even if this results in a slight decrease in levels of local control. The proven ability to salvage radiotherapy failures using multi-agent aggressive chemotherapy is certainly playing a role in the willingness to explore the deliberate under-dosing of sensitive tissues at risk. Reliable sets of data demonstrating actual improvements in outcomes using these techniques have not yet appeared in the literature and are anxiously awaited by the oncology world.

Radioimmunotherapy for Low-grade B-cell non-Hodgkin's Lymphoma

Since NHL in general, and low-grade B-cell NHL in particular, are generally disseminated at the time of presentation, it is reasonable to assume that systemic treatments such as chemotherapy are likely to play dominant roles in disease management. With the convincing documentation that antibody-based therapeutics, such as the chimeric antibody Rituximab, produce high response rates for low-grade B-cell NHL and that these response rates can be further improved by the addition of chemotherapy, it became clear that antibody-based immunotherapeutic treatments directed against highly expressed cell surface antigens such as CD20 deserved serious consideration in the development of multi-modality management strategies for both low grade and higher grade B-cell NHL [15]. Unfortunately, the clinical responses to anti-CD20 agents such as Rituximab are often incomplete and of short duration. This is especially true for aggressive B-cell cases, which may have relapsed multiple times after intensive cyotoxic chemotherapy. The addition of rituximab to conventional chemotherapy regimens has produced increased RFS and OS for many types of B-cell NHL. Unfortunately, curative strategies remain elusive. For this reason, it seemed reasonable to consider ways to "turbo charge" antibodies and other biological therapeutics to increase effectiveness against this responsive disease group. For antibody-based therapy, one mechanism being explored in this effort involves the use of radiolabeled antibodies directed at the same CD20 surface antigen that serves as a target for rituximab. The first FDA-cleared therapeutic radiolabeled antibody, Y-90 Ibritumomab Tiuxetan ("Zevalin"), first appeared in 2002, followed 1 year later by I-131 radiolabeled Tositumomab ("Bexxar") [16].

Both of these compounds produced excellent response rates and were approved for the treatment of refractory, relapsed and transformed CD20-positive B-cell NHL (See Fig. 6.1). It is notable that for both Y-90 Zevalin and for I-131 Bexxar, patients with bulky disease produce less durable responses to treatment. Patterns of recurrence from the Cleveland Clinic, now confirmed at other sites, show that bulky disease sites appear to relapse more often and faster than non-bulky disease sites in patients treated with Y-90 Zevalin (Fig. 6.1). Clinical trials evaluating the use of external beam radiotherapy combined with anti-CD20 RIT are underway in an attempt to cytoreduce the bulky disease sites and eliminate the unfavorable risk profile associated with this disease characteristic (See Fig. 6.2). Figure 2 depicts a graph showing progression free survival vs overall survival in patients with relapsed or refractory bulky follicular lymphoma treated with external beam radiation therapy followed by yttrium-90 ibritumomab tiuxetan from a recent trial at our center [17].

REFERENCES

1. Z Chustecka. Non-Hodgkin lymphoma survival has increased over past decade. Arch Intern Med 168:469–76, 2008.
2. RW Tsang, M Gospodarowicz, J Yahalom. Low-grade non Hodgkin lymphomas: seminars in radiation oncology. Lymphoma 17:198, 2007.
3. PM Peterson, M Gospodarowicz, R Tsang, et al. Long-term outcome in stage I and II follicular lymphoma following treatment with involved field radiation therapy alone. J Clin Oncol 22:563, 2004.
4. CS HA, F Cabanillas, M-S Lee, et al. Serial determination of the bcl-2 gene in the bone marrow and peripheral blood after central lymphatic irradiation for stages I–III follicular lymphoma: a preliminary report. Clin Cancer Res 3:215–19, 1997.
5. JO Armitage, DD Weisenburger. New approach to classifying non-Hodgkin's lymphomas: clinical features of the major histologic sub-types. Non-Hodgkin's Lymphoma Classification Project. J Clin Oncol 16:2780–95, 1998.
6. M Mac Manus, RT Hoppe. Is radiotherapy curative for stage I and II low-grade follicular lymphoma? Results of a long-term follow-up study of patients treated at Standford University. J Clin Oncol 14:1282–90, 1996.
7. B Vaughan Hudson, G Vaughan Hudson, KA MacLennan, et al. Clinical stage 1 non-Hodgkin's lymphoma: long-term follow-up of patients treated by the British National Lymphoma Investigation with radiotherapy alone as initial therapy. Br J Cancer 69:1088–93, 1994.
8. AM Kirby, NG Mikhaeel. The role of FDG PET in the management of lymphoma: what is the evidence base? Nucl Med Commun 28(5):335–54, 2007.
9. BA Guadagnolo, S Li, D Neuberg, et al. Long-term outcome and mortality trends in early-stage, Grade 1-2 follicular lymphoma treated with radiation therapy. Int J Radiat Oncol Biol Phys 64:928–34, 2006.
10. RW Tsang, M Gospodarowicz, J Yahalom. Low-grade non Hodgkin lymphomas: seminars in radiation oncology. Lymphoma 17:198, 2007.
11. PM Richard, P Soubeyran, H Eghbali, et al. Place of low-dose total body irradiation in the treatment of localized follicular

non-Hodgkin's lymphoma: results of a pilot study. Int J Radiat Oncol Bio Phys 40(2):387–90, 1998.

12. T Girinsky, M Ghalibafian. Radiotherapy of Hodgkin lymphoma: indications. New fields, and techniques. Semin Radiat Oncol 17:206–22, 2007.

13. L Specht. 2-(18F) Fluoro-2-deoxyglucose positron-emission tomography in staging, response evaluation, and treatment planning of lymphomas. Semin Radiat Oncol 17:190–97, 2007.

14. T Grinsky, C Pichenot, A Beaudre. Is intensity-modulated radiotherapy better than conventional radiation treatment and three-conformal radiotherapy for mediastinal masses in patients with Hodgkin disease, and is there a role for beam orientation optimization and dose constraints assigned to virtual volumes? Int J Radiat Oncol Biol Phys 64:218–26, 2006.

15. RM Macklis. Radioimmunotherapy as a therapeutic option for non-Hodgkin's lymphoma. Semin Radiat Oncol 17:176–83, 2007.

16. BL Pohlman, JW Sweetenham, RM Macklis. Review of clinical radioimmunotherapy. Expert Rev Anticancer Ther 22:445–62, 2006.

17. M Burdick, R Macklis. External Beam Radiotherapy Followed by 90Y Ibritumomab Tiuxetan in Relapsed or Refractory Bulky Follicular Lymphoma. Int J Radiat Oncol Biol Phys. 2010. [Epub ahead of print]

7 Aggressive B-Cell Non-Hodgkin's Lymphoma
Henry Blair and Nidhi Sharma

CHAPTER SUMMARY

Although both radiotherapy (RT) and chemotherapy can produce impressive responses in patients with localized diffuse large B-cell (DLBC) non-Hodgkin's lymphoma (NHL), the modern era has witnessed a gradual increase in importance for systemic chemotherapy and a corresponding decrease in importance for RT. This trend results in large part from the recognition that aggressive NHL is a systemic disease and may be effectively controlled and in many cases cured using current multi-agent systemic regimens such as CHOP (cyclophosphamide, doxorubicin, vincristine and prednisone), whereas wide-field RT regimens often produce only temporary remissions. Thus, the standard of care for virtually all cases of aggressive lymphoma (including subtypes such as DLBC NHL) require systemic treatment, with RT used only selectively for consolidation or palliation. The development of anti-CD20 immunotherapy, including the chimeric monoclonal antibody rituximab, appears to be adding substantially to tumor control rates and this agent has now been incorporated into many standard treatment paradigms for both early- and late-stage DLBC NIIL. Thus, systemic treatments have clearly assumed the primary role in multimodality management approaches for aggressive NHL, with likely outcomes and optimal treatment intensity often selected in reference to the International Prognostic Index (IPI), a prognostic scoring system most broadly validated for systemically treated aggressive B-cell lymphoma [1], and is discussed below.

RT may still play major roles in consolidation after chemotherapy, but concerns about radiotoxicity have resulted in a major trend toward limitation of RT fields and doses. Newer technologies, such as intensity-modulated RT (IMRT) and image-guided RT (IGRT), allow the use of highly conformal dose delivery patterns, and the recent incorporation of functional imaging studies, such as ^{18}F-fluorodeoxyglucose-positron emission tomography ([^{18}F]FDG-PET), allows treatment fields and doses to be tailored to the extent and response patterns of individual cases. A key principle emerging in the current era thus appears to be risk-adjusted combination therapies with minimal delayed organ toxicity and secondary tumor risks. Immunotherapeutics such as rituximab appear to be powerful new additions to the armamentarium of systemic treatment regimen for B-cell NHL.

Introduction and Background

DLBCL is the most common lymphoid malignancy in adults with approximately 25,000 cases per year in the USA. This represents about 30% of total NHL [2,3]. The median age is 70–80 years. Patients often present with a history of an enlarging lymph node, in 40% of patients the site is extranodal. Up to a third of the patients have stage IV disease. Bone marrow is involved in 15% patients. Another third of the patients have systemic "B" symptoms. Half have elevated serum lactate dehydrogenase (LDH) [4]. It is also the most common histology of extranodal NHL [4].

Classification Systems

The histopathologic classification systems developed for lymphoid malignancies continue to be revised as newly acquired information results in greater consensus among the experts, and have changed several times since the initial system (Rappaport) in 1966. The nomenclature for DLBCL is shown in Table A.1 [5].

The WHO classification used morphology, immunophenotype, cytogenetic and molecular features and clinical behavior in the definition of each disease subtype [6]. DLBCL has different clinical patterns of presentation and behavior including: primary mediastinal, intravascular and primary effusion lymphomas [7]. Primary mediastinal (thymic) large B-cell lymphoma (MLBCL) is often described as a localized, sclerotic mass in young female patients [8].

Prognostic Indices

Aggressive NHL is a dangerous and potentially lethal disease. It warrants the adjective "aggressive" [9] as untreated survival figures on the order of just 1–2 years are common. Historically, the Ann Arbor staging system was developed for Hodgkin's disease [1] and subsequently applied to both Hodgkin's lymphoma (HL) and NHL. There is variability in survival and response curves within the same Ann Arbor stage for NHL. In order to develop an index/model to predict overall survival (OS) and relapse-free survival in patients with aggressive NHL on the basis of the patients' clinical characteristics, the International Non-Hodgkin's Lymphoma Prognostic Factors Project was undertaken. In 1993 [1], a collection of 2031 adult patients with aggressive histology, submitted by 16 institutions in the USA, Europe and Canada, treated between 1982 and 1987 with combination chemotherapy regimens containing doxorubicin, were analyzed for clinical features to create this index.

Statistical analysis of this data (Appendix A) resulted in a combination of age, Ann Arbor stage, number of extranodal sites of disease, performance status and LDH as significant prognostic factors and four risk groups (Table A.2) with predicted 5-year survival rates of 73, 51, 43 and 26% were created. Analysis for patients ≤60 (1274 patients) [1] is depicted in Table A.3. Sixty years was chosen as a break point due to the exclusion age for most protocols at that time.

For patients older than 60 years, the 5-year survival rates were as shown in Table A.4. The international index and the age-adjusted international index were significantly more accurate than the Ann Arbor classification in predicting long-term survival.

Limited or Early-stage Disease

Most of the patients with limited disease by IPI criteria (stage I–II, one or no sites of extranodal disease and typically better than poor performance status) can be classified as low-risk IPI unless they are >60 years, have elevated serum LDH or poor performance status, yet can have widely varying results to similar treatment.

Table 7.1 Adverse Risk Factors, as Defined by the IPI, Refined for Use in Patients with Limited Disease

Adverse risk factor	IPI	Stage-modified IPI
Stage	III, IV	Non-bulky
Age	>60	>60
LDH	> Normal	> Normal
PS	≥2	≥2
"E" sites	≥2	Not applicable

IPI, International Prognostic Index; LDH, lactate dehydrogenase, PS, performance status; E, extranodal.

Miller et al. proposed a modified IPI for patients with limited disease [10] (Table 7.1) and claimed that patients with no adverse risk factors have a 5-year survival of 94%, while patients with three or four adverse risk factors have a poor 5-year survival of only 50%.

Measuring Response to Treatment

Methods to document and measure response after treatment include physical examination, imaging studies, serum chemistry tests and biopsies. Computed tomography (CT) scans have replaced lymphangiography, gallium scanning and staging laparotomy and PET/CT scans can add prognostic information after two cycles of chemotherapy. Spaepen et al. [11] reviewed [18F]FDG-PET scans in 70 patients with aggressive NHL (majority with DLBCL) treated with doxorubicin-containing chemotherapy. PET scans were taken prior to the start of treatment and at mid-treatment. None of the 33 patients with persistent abnormal [18F]FDG uptake at mid-treatment achieved a durable complete remission (CR) versus 31/37 patients with a negative scan who remained in CR with a median follow-up of 1107 days. Furthermore, a multivariate analysis showed [18F]FDG-PET at mid-treatment was a stronger prognostic factor for progression-free survival (PFS) ($p < 1 \times 10^{-7}$) and OS ($p < 9 \times 10^{-6}$) than IPI ($p < 0.11$ and $p < 0.03$, respectively).

In an effort to establish a consensus on a standardized set of guidelines for response assessment in adult patients with indolent and aggressive NHL after treatment, the National Cancer Institute (NCI) sponsored two workshops (February and May 1998) and their recommendations were published in 1999 [12]. A lymph node >1 cm in its longest transverse diameter was interpreted to be involved with NHL, and CT scans were qualified as the "standard" for evaluation of nodal disease. The significance of a residual abdominal mass is particularly problematic as 30–50% of patients with a large intra-abdominal mass at presentation and for whom the physical examination is normal after therapy will have a residual mass [12]. A review of 241 patients [13] with aggressive lymphoma treated at the NCI from 1977 to 1986 found 29 patients had radiologically stable residual masses after therapy, and of 22 (76%) with pathologic evaluations, 21 had negative specimens (95%) and one was positive (5%) with no relapse in the abdominal site at 31 months after follow-up in patients with negative pathologic evaluation.

[18F]FDG-PET technology is based on observations in the 1920s by Professor Otto Warburg, 1931 Nobel Prize Winner in Physiology or Medicine, that cancer cells accumulate glucose (as FDG-6-phosphate) in higher intracellular amounts than non-malignant cells. In 1987, [18F]FDG-PET planar imaging was shown to be more avid than [67Ga] citrate in five patients with NHL [14]. In December 2000, the Centers for Medicare and Medicaid Services (CMS) gave Medicare coverage for the use of PET for non-small cell lung cancer, esophageal cancer, colorectal cancer, lymphoma, melanoma, head and neck cancers (excluding thyroid) and limited coverage for myocardial viability, and the indications continue to expand. For NHL, the overall sensitivity of [18F]FDG-PET imaging versus CT is approximately 15% higher (90 vs. 75%, respectively), whereas the specificity is the same for both imaging modalities (100%) [15].

As the resolution of PET scanners improved and clinical protocols proliferated, to help standardize the acquisition and interpretation of [18F]-FDG-PET images in clinical trials sponsored by the NCI, the Cancer Imaging Program of the NCI convened a workshop on January 10–11, 2005, in Washington, DC [17].

They adopted the technical guidelines of Shankar [16] for PET scans:

1. Patients should fast for at least 4 hours prior to the FDG injection.
2. Blood glucose level should not exceed 200 mg/dL (11 mmol/L) at the time of FDG injection. Re-schedule FDG-PET and attempt to control the blood sugar level if blood glucose level exceeds this level.
3. Encompass at least the region between the base of the skull and the mid-thigh in two- or three-dimensional mode.
4. FDG dose of 3.5–8 MBq/kg of body weight, with a minimum dose of 185 MBq in adults (5 mCi) and 18.5 MBq (0.5 mCi) in children.
5. Whole-body imaging should begin 50–70 minutes after the administration of FDG.
6. The PET projection data should be corrected for random coincidences, scatter and attenuation in accordance with manufacturer's recommendations.
7. The reconstructed PET or PET/CT images must be displayed on a computer workstation so that transaxial, sagittal and coronal images can be viewed simultaneously.
8. Although CT standards and technology continue to evolve, some general principles should be adopted for all studies. Contrast enhancement in the arterial and/or portal venous phase is essential at initial staging and for follow-up studies whenever hepatic or splenic involvement was documented previously.
9. Oral contrast material should also be administered to optimize differentiation of bowel from other abdominopelvic structures.
10. Multi-detector CT technology will minimize scan time and maximize anatomic coverage.

Their recommendations regarding the use of PET scans included [17]:

1. PET after completion of therapy should be performed at least 3 weeks, preferably at 6–8 weeks, after chemotherapy or chemoimmunotherapy, and 8–12 weeks after radiation or chemoradiotherapy.
2. Visual assessment alone is adequate for interpreting PET findings as positive or negative when assessing response after completion of therapy.

3. Mediastinal blood pool activity is recommended as the reference background activity to define PET positivity for a residual mass ≥2 cm in greatest transverse diameter, regardless of its location. A smaller residual mass or a normal-sized lymph node (i.e., ≤1×1 cm in diameter) should be considered positive if its activity is above that of the surrounding background.
4. Use of attenuation-corrected PET is strongly encouraged.
5. Use of PET for treatment monitoring during a course of therapy should only be done in a clinical trial or as part of a prospective registry.

Newer Treatment Options

Rituximab was approved by the Food and Drug Administration on November 26, 1997, for the indication of relapsed or refractory, CD-20 positive, B-cell, low-grade or follicular NHL [18]. Subsequent trials of Rituximab and CHOP (anthracylcine-based) in diffuse large cell lymphoma (DLCL) showed R-CHOP (Rituxan+CHOP) was superior to CHOP alone in both low-risk and high-risk patients, in patients aged 60–70 or 70–80 years [19], in younger patients (aged 18–60 years) and patients who had no risk factors or one risk factor according to age-adjusted IPI, stage II–IV disease or bulky stage I disease [22]. The IPI was developed prior to the introduction of Rituxan.

New chemotherapy agents are continually being created, studied and administered either as single agents or part of a multi-drug regimen (e.g., EPOCH: etoposide, vincristine and doxorubicin with bolus doses of cyclophosphamide and oral prednisone plus rituximab versus CHOP plus rituximab) [20]. Biotherapies such as immunotherapy are now beginning to play important roles as well. Recently, data have emerged from multiple sites testifying to the importance and effectiveness of anti-CD20 immunotherapy (such as the chimeric antibody rituximab) in conjunction with chemotherapy for the management of this patient group. In comparison to systemic therapeutics, local field RT is now playing a much smaller role than in the past for aggressive lymphoma [19,21,22]. This is despite the clear cellular sensitivity of this histology to cell death induced by ionizing radiation. The use of radiation attached to monoclonal antibodies (radioimmunotherapy; RIT) may represent a potential "quantum leap" in the use of ionizing radiation against lymphoma.

Typical Radiation Therapy Doses for Aggressive Lymphoma

Nieder et al. [23] reviewed papers published from 1990 to 2003 regarding radiation therapy dose and recommended the following minimum doses for involved-field RT:

1. Initial size <3.5 cm (possibly <6 cm) with CR after chemotherapy can be treated with 30 or 30.6 Gy
2. The next group might be sufficiently controlled by 36 Gy, but it remains unclear whether the cut-off should be 6 cm or higher
3. 7–10 cm: 40 Gy. Most likely, 45 Gy does not have to be exceeded for larger lesions

Although, essentially, all lymphoma subtypes exhibit at least moderate radio-responsiveness, it does appear that some types are more sensitive to very low-dose treatment and some require higher dose levels. Aggressive lymphoma subtypes are traditionally thought to require doses on the order of 40–55 Gy, whereas more sensitive histologies, such as low-grade B-cell NHL and HL, may be controlled in doses ranging from 20 to 40 Gy. When used as a component of a multimodality regimen for aggressive NHL, it appears that doses of approximately 30–36 Gy are appropriate for the local control of microscopic disease and doses of approximately 40–45 Gy are indicated for residual gross disease sites.

Based upon a review of the medical literature, Wirth's [24] recommendations for the use of RT with R-CHOP for DLBCL are as shown in Table 7.2.

Table 7.2 Recommendations for Use of Radiotherapy with R-CHOP for DLBCL[24]

Setting	Recommendation	Comments
Stage I–II without risk factors	R-CHOP×3+IFRT	Expect primarily 90% freedom from progression, long-term follow-up data available (for CHOP×3+RT)
	R-CHOP×6 alone	Comparable outcome anticipated, but long-term data unavailable – consider when IFRT poses unacceptable morbidity risk*
Stage I–II with bulky disease	R-CHOP×6+IFRT	May withhold IFRT if unacceptable morbidity risk*
Extranodal primary site	R-CHOP×6+CNS prophylaxis, with IFRT to contralateral testis and consider IFRT to initially involved nodes	
CNS	High-dose methotrexate regimen. Consider cranial RT for patients <60	Patients <60 generally should receive chemotherapy alone
Bone, breast	R-CHOP×6+IFRT	
Head and neck	R-CHOP×6+IFRT	Consider withholding IFRT if extensive salivary gland morbidity cannot be avoided even with optimal radiotherapy planning
Mediastinum	R-CHOP×6+IFRT	
Other site	Apply general principles for stage I–II	Available data inconclusive, may withhold IFRT if unacceptable morbidity risk*
Stage III–IV	R-CHOP×6+IFRT to bulky site	May withhold IFRT if unacceptable morbidity risk*

*Unacceptable morbidity risk: cases where IFRT leads to significant breast exposure in women age <30, or extensive cardiac, pulmonary, salivary or other critical organ exposure that cannot be avoided with suitable planning techniques.

Outside of a clinical trial for frontline therapy, the major role for RT is to decrease relapse in the irradiated field [25,26]. It should be noted, the Groupe d'Etude des Lymphomes de l'Adulte (GELA) wrote in 2007 "the GELA decided to abandon radiotherapy as first-line treatment of localized aggressive lymphoma, with the advantage of avoiding its late effects, especially in the frequently involved cervical and Waldeyer's ring regions" [26]. As called for by Ng and Mauch in their 2007 editorial: "To meaningfully clarify the role of radiation therapy in localized aggressive lymphoma, the most informative trial will be one that employs CHOP and rituximab, followed by either radiation therapy using modern technique or no additional therapy" [27].

Radiation Therapy for Early-stage Aggressive NHL

An important set of early studies on consolidative radiation therapy (XRT) for early-stage aggressive NHL is represented by the data in two randomized trials from the 1990s, both designed to explore the question of whether RT was a meaningful contributor to an integrated management strategy. SWOG 8736 [28] enrolled patients with stage I, IE, II and IIE with biopsy-proved, intermediate- or high-grade NHL (working-formulation groups D through J). They were randomly assigned to receive either three cycles of CHOP followed by involved-field RT (IFRT) (200 patients) to a dose of 40–55 Gy versus eight cycles of CHOP without any XRT (201 patients). At the 5-year period (paper published in 1998), PFS (77%) and OS (72%) were both significantly improved over chemotherapy alone (PFS and OS: 64 and 72%, respectfully). An important caveat is the gradually decreasing significance of the difference over time, as demonstrated on subsequent updates and

the fact that much or all of the survival advantage may have been due to excess cardiac mortality getting eight full cycles of CHOP chemotherapy [10].

ECOG 1484 (published 2004) compared 30-Gy RT with observation in stage I with mediastinal or retroperitoneal involvement or bulky disease >10 cm in diameter, and stage IE, II or IIE adults (>16 years) with diffuse aggressive lymphoma in complete response after eight cycles of CHOP [25]. Partial response (PR) patients received 40-Gy RT. No survival differences were observed. Three patients treated with radiation therapy versus 15 patients not treated with radiation therapy relapsed in initial disease sites. At 6 years, failure-free survival was 63% in PR patients; conversion to CR did not significantly influence clinical outcome.

Two similar studies were carried out by the GELA group. The LNH-93-1 study randomized low-risk patients age <60 to either three cycles of intensive ACVPB followed by chemotherapy consolidation versus three cycles of CHOP followed by IFRT (30–40 Gy). The event-free survival (EFS) and OS were significantly improved in the intensive chemotherapy group, though most relapses in the chemotherapy alone group showed a pattern of recurrence involving the original disease site.

Patients aged over 60 years with low-risk disease were randomized to either four cycles of CHOP alone versus four cycles of CHOP followed by 40-Gy radiation therapy. No significant difference was noted in EFS (68 vs. 66%) or OS (68 vs. 72%).

Ng [29] and Wirth [24] reviewed the published studies of radiation therapy in early-stage aggressive lymphoma (Table 7.3).

For all these studies, a key weakness in using this data to inform current treatment decisions relates to the time period in which

Table 7.3 Randomized Trials of Chemotherapy Alone Versus Chemotherapy and Radiation Therapy in Limited-Stage DBCL [37]

Study	Patient population	No.	Medical follow up period (in years)	Treatment arms	Results	ρ Value
SWOG 8736[28]	Stage I or IE (bulky and non-bulky); stage II or IIE (non-bulky only)	401	4.4 year	CHOP×3 then 40–55 Gy IFRT versus CHOP×8 alone	5-year PFS: 77%	0.03
					5-year OS: 92%	0.02
					5-year PFS: 64%	
					5-year OS: 72%	
ECOG 1484[25]	Stage I (bulky or EN only); stage II (bulky and non-bulky)	215 (172 randomized)	12 years	CHOP×8: if CR then randomize between 30 Gy IFRT versus no RT	6-year DFS: 69%	0.05
				If PR, then 40 Gy IFRT	6-year FFS: 70%	0.05
					6-year OS: 79%	0.23
					6-year DFS: 53%	
					6-year FFS: 53%	
					6-year OS: 67%	
					6-year FFS: 63%	
					6-year OS: 69%	
LNH-93-1[30]	Age <60 (10% bulky, 50% EN, 0 aaIPI)	647	7.7 year	ACVBP then MTX, ifosfamide, VP16, Ara-C versus CHOP×3 then if RT 30–40 Gy	5-year EFS: 82%	0.004
					5-year OS: 90%	0.001
					5-year EFS: 74%	
					5-year OS: 81%	
LNH-93-4[26]	Age <60 (8% bulky; 56% EN)	576	6.8 year	CHOP×4 then if RT 40 Gy versus CHOP×4	EFS: 66%	0.7
					OS: 72%	0.6
					EFS: 68%	
					OS: 68%	

the studies were performed – the pre-rituximab era. We do not yet have convincing comprehensive data evaluating limited chemotherapy (e.g., three cycles of CHOP) plus rituximab to a similar regimen followed by XFRT. Such a trial is urgently needed to understand the role of XRT in the management of limited-stage DLBC NHL in the era of rituximab and risk-adjusted treatment regimens.

The Southwest Oncology Group study (SWOG 0014 published in 2008) [31] is a phase II trial of aggressive, CD20-expressing NHL, including DLBCL, mantle-cell lymphoma, Burkitt's or Burkitt-like lymphoma and B-cell phenotype of anaplastic large-cell lymphoma with (limited stage) stage I, IE or non-bulky II or IIE disease by Ann Arbor classification. Bulky disease was defined as any mass exceeding 10 cm in maximal diameter, or a mediastinal mass with a maximal diameter exceeding one-third of maximal chest diameter. Patients also had to have at least one adverse risk factor as defined by the stage-modified IPI (non-bulky stage II disease, age >60 years, WHO performance status of 2 or elevated serum LDH). Limited-disease patients with no adverse risk factors (stage I, younger age, normal serum LDH and good performance status) were excluded from the trial because their OS was 95–97% at 5 years [28,32]. Fifty-seven patients (95%) received radiation therapy.

Fifty-one of 54 patients (95%) completed radiation therapy at planned dosage (40–55 Gy). Most of the patients (91%) received doses in the range of 40–46 Gy. The median dose delivered was 41.4 Gy. Radiation therapy was initiated at a median of 24 days after administration of intravenous CHOP chemotherapy.

All but two patients began radiation therapy before Day 35. Sixty patients with aggressive NHL were eligible. With the median follow-up of 5.3 years, treatment resulted in a PFS of 93% at 2 years and 88% at 4 years. OS was 95% at 2 years and 92% at 4 years. The authors compared these results with those from a historic group of patients treated without rituximab on SWOG 8736 (PFS of 78% and OS of 88% at 4 years) and interpreted their results as showing a benefit.

For advanced stage and recurrent disease, radiotherapy plans are individualized and often the chosen regimens are dictated by patients' symptoms, pattern of disease progression and other simultaneously planned treatment therapies. The role of stem-cell transplant (either autologous or allageneic) is currently being defined. In these cases, the incentive to limit the volume of tissue exposed to high-dose RT is readily apparent. In some studies, PET/CT (positron emission technology scan fused with a CT scan) metabolic imaging has shown the change in metabolic activity (reported as standardized uptake value; SUV) after one or two cycles of chemotherapy and this change can predict the success of the treatment and may ultimately be used to allow adaptive dosing. Data for this approach are not yet widely available.

Radiation therapy can be offered to patients who fail CHOP or R-CHOP as part of their salvage regimen with high-dose therapy and autologous stem-cell rescue. Hoppe et al. [33] reviewed the effectiveness of IFRT in 164 patients with relapsed or refractory DLCL before high-dose chemotherapy and autologous stem-cell rescue. IFRT was delivered to involved sites measuring >5 cm or to sites with residual disease >2 cm. The dose was 30 Gy delivered in 1.5-Gy fractions twice daily. Median follow-up was 60 months.

Two- and five-year PFS was 62 and 53%; two- and five-year OS was 67 and 58%, respectively.

Influence of Bulk

"Bulky" disease usually refers to hilar or mediastinal disease and previous definitions include: size <7.5 cm, size <10 cm, size greater than one-third transthoracic diameter in different studies.

From 1989 to 1997, Aviles et al. [34] enrolled 166 patients with IPI intermediate-high to high. Eight-two were randomized to radiation therapy (30 Gy) and 84 randomized to observation. PET scans were not available. Eligibility criteria included: age <18 years to <70 years; previously treated with an anthracycline-based regimen: CHOP or CEOP (epirubicin 90 mg/m², instead of doxorubicin); presence after six cycles of residual mass (<5 cm); negative for immunodeficiency virus. They reported (2005) with median follow-up of 135 months, actuarial curves at 10 years showed: progressive-free disease: 86% in patients treated with salvage radiation versus 32% in the unirradiated group ($p<0.001$) and OS: 89% in patients treated with salvage radiation versus 58% in the unirradiated group ($p<0.001$).

The MabThera International Trial (MInT) Group(ref 35) randomly assigned 823 young individuals aged 18–60 years, from 18 countries with good-prognosis (none or one risk factor according to the age-adjusted [aa]-IPI, stages II–IV or stage I with bulky disease) DLBCL to six cycles of CHOP-like chemotherapy with or without rituximab. Tumor masses (single lymph nodes or conglomerates) with a diameter (i.e., MTD) of more than or equal to 5.0 cm, more than or equal to 7.5 cm, or more than or equal to 10.0 cm, were defined as bulky disease according to the cut-off point pre-defined by each cooperative group. RT to primary extranodal disease was given to 52 patients at the physician's discretion and the doses ranged from 30 to 40 Gy. Response was assessed on day 155 after starting treatment, according to the International Workshop criteria. Of the patients, 28% had tumor bulk <5.0 cm and did not receive radiation therapy. Only 3% of the patients had bulky disease ≥10.0 cm.

For patients receiving CHOP-like treatment, any cut-off point between 5.0 and 10.0 cm separated two populations with significant EFS difference ($p<0.0001$ for all log-rank tests) and OS difference ($p≤0.003$ for all log-rank tests). For CHOP-like chemotherapy and rituximab, only a cut-off point of 10.0 cm separated two populations with a significant EFS difference (log-rank $p=0.047$), but any cut-off point of 6.0 cm or more separated two populations with a significant OS difference (log-rank p values 0.0009–0.037).

Radioimmunotherapy for Aggressive B-cell non-Hodgkin's Lymphoma

Zinzani et al. [36] reported the results of prospective, single-arm, open-label, non-randomized phase II combination chemotherapy with CHOP plus RIT trial in untreated, elderly, diffuse large B-cell lymphoma (DLBCL) patients. Twenty eligible patients (age range: 60–84 years) with previously untreated DLBCL received six cycles of CHOP chemotherapy followed 6–10 weeks later by 90Y ibritumomab tiuxetan. The overall response rate was 100%, including 95% CR and 5% partial remission. Four (80%) of the five patients who achieved less than a CR with CHOP improved their remission status after RIT. With a median follow-up of 15 months, the

2-year PFS was estimated to be 75%, with a 2-year OS of 95%. The role of such systemic radiopharmaceutical treatment will be clarified as clinical trial data mature.

Principles of Image-guided Radiotherapy Techniques for Aggressive B-cell non-Hodgkin's Lymphoma Management

At present, there are few technical reports in the literature on the use of IGRT specifically for aggressive NHL. Therefore, we must apply the principles described for general NHL management incorporating IGRT for field design and treatment. As summarized in Chapter 1, the main principles would include the following:

1. Both pre-treatment and post-treatment PET or PET/CT should be obtained for patients undergoing chemotherapy regimens prior to receiving radiation therapy. Treatment planning considerations include factors such as: the apparent degree of involvement of all clinically involved nodal and extended groups, the degree and rapidity of response to chemotherapy, the proximity of nearby critical normal tissues and the presence of post-chemotherapy residual FDG-avid tissues or FDG-negative "scar" tissue demonstrated on CT or MRI.
2. Deliberately inhomogeneous dose delivery strategies with IMRT methodologies where warranted by normal tissue proximity will result in highly conformal dose delivery with minimization of normal tissue margins.
3. Appropriate immobilization using templates, masks, positioning rigs, etc.
4. Serial re-evaluation during the course of treatment to determine whether registration coordinates have moved or if "adaptive" re-planning or re-calculation of absorbed doses is warranted.

As correlative data utilizing FDG-PET and the results of modern integrated multimodality therapy appear in the literature, it will be increasingly simple to develop a unified management consensus.

At present, the role of RT in the management of aggressive histologies such as DLBCL is in flux and wide variations in individual practice patterns will continue to be the rule.

REFERENCES

1. A predictive model for aggressive non-Hodgkin's lymphoma. The International Non-Hodgkin's Lymphoma Prognostic Factors Project. N J Engl Med 329:987–94, 1993.
2. JO Armitage, DD Weisenburger. New approach to classifying non-Hodgkin's lymphomas: clinical features of the major histologic subtypes. Non-Hodgkin's Lymphoma Classification Project. J Clin Oncol 16:2780–95, 1998.
3. LM Morton, SS Wang, SS Devesa, et al. Lymphoma incidence patterns by WHO subtype in the United States, 1992–2001. Blood 107:265–76, 2006.
4. KE Hunt, KK Reichard. Diffuse large B-cell lymphoma. Arch Pathol Lab Med 132:118–24, 2008.
5. JA Abramson, MA Shipp. Advances in the biology and therapy of diffuse large B-cell lymphoma: moving toward a molecularly targeted approach. Blood 106:1164–74, 2005.
6. ES Jaffe, NL Harris, H Stein, et al. (eds) World Health Organization classification of tumours. Pathology and genetics of tumours of haematopoietic and lymphoid tissues. Lyon: IARC Press; 2001.
7. KC Gatter, RA Warnke. Diffuse large B-cell lymphoma. In: ES Jaffe, NL Harris, H Stein, JW Vardiman (eds) World Health Organization classification of tumours pathology and genetics of tumours of haematopoietic and lymphoid tissues. Lyon: IARC Press 171–74, 2001.
8. KJ Savage, S Monti, JL Kutok, et al. The molecular signature of mediastinal large B-cell lymphoma differs from that of other diffuse large B cell lymphomas and shares features with classical Hodgkin lymphoma. Blood 102:3871–79, 2003.
9. AC Aisenberg. Coherent view of non-Hodgkin's lymphoma. J Clin Oncol 23:2656–75, 1995.
10. TP Miller, CM Spier, L Rimsza. Diffuse aggressive histologies of non-Hodgkin lymphoma: treatment and biology of limited disease. Semin Hematol 43:207–12, 2006.
11. K Spaepen, S Stroobants, P Dupont, et al. Early restaging positron emission tomography with (18)F-fluorodeoxyglucose predicts outcome in patients with aggressive non-Hodgkin's lymphoma. Ann Oncol 13:1356–63, 2002.
12. BD Cheson, SJ Horning, B Coiffier, et al. Report of an international workshop to standardize response criteria for non-Hodgkin's lymphoma. NCI Sponsored International Working Group. J Clin Oncol 17:1244, 1999.
13. A Surbone, DL Longo, VT Jr DeVita, et al. Residual abdominal masses in aggressive non-Hodgkin's lymphoma after combination chemotherapy: significance and management. J Clin Oncol 6:1832–37, 1988.
14. R Paul. Comparison of fluorine-18-2-fluorodeoxyglucose and gallium-67 citrate imaging for detection of lymphoma. J Nucl Med 28:288–92, 1987.
15. C Schiepers. PET for staging of Hodgkin's disease and non-Hodgkin's lymphoma. J Eur Nucl Med Mol Imaging 30(Suppl. 1):S82–S88, 2003.
16. M Juweid. Use of positron emission tomography for response assessment of lymphoma: consensus of the Imaging Subcommittee of International Harmonization Project in Lymphoma. J Clin Oncol 25:571–78, 2007.
17. LK Shankar, JM Hoffman, S Bacharach, et al. Consensus recommendations for the use of FDG PET as indicator of therapeutic response in patients in National Cancer Institute trials. J Nucl Med 47:1059–66, 2006.
18. AJ Grillo-Lopez, CA White, C Varns, et al. Overview of the clinical development of rituximab: first monoclonal antibody approved for the treatment of lymphoma. Semin Oncol 26(5 Suppl 14):66–73, 1999.
19. B Coiffier, E Lepage, J Briere, et al. CHOP chemotherapy plus Rituximab compared with CHOP alone in elderly patients with diffuse large B-cell lymphoma. N J Engl Med 346: 235–42, 2002.
20. W Wilson, K Dunleavy, S Pittaluga, et al. Phase II study of dose-adjusted EPOCH and Rituximab in untreated diffuse large B-cell lymphoma with analysis of germinal center and post-germinal center biomarkers. J Clin Oncol 26: 2717–24, 2008.

21. TM Habermann, EA Weller, VA Morrison, et al. Rituximab-CHOP versus CHOP alone or with maintenance rituximab in older patients with diffuse large B-cell lymphoma. J Clin Oncol 24:3121–27, 2006.

22. M Pfreundschuh, L Trumper, A Osterborg, et al. CHOP-like chemotherapy plus rituximab versus CHOP-like chemotherapy alone in young patients with good-prognosis diffuse large-B-cell lymphoma: a randomised controlled trial by the MabThera International Trial (MInT) Group. Lancet Oncol 7:379–91, 2006.

23. C Nieder, T Licht, N Andratschke, et al. Influence of differing radiotherapy strategies on treatment results in diffuse large-cell lymphoma: a review. Cancer Treat Rev 29:11–19, 2003.

24. A Wirth. The rationale and role of radiation therapy in the treatment of patients with diffuse large B-cell lymphoma in the Rituximab era. Leuk Lymphoma 48:2121–36, 2007.

25. SJ Horning, E Weller, K Kim, et al. Chemotherapy with or without radiotherapy in limited-stage diffuse aggressive non-Hodgkin's lymphoma: Eastern Cooperative Oncology Group study 1484. J Clin Oncol 22:3032–38, 2004.

26. C Bonnet, G Fillet, N Mounier, et al. CHOP alone compared with CHOP plus radiotherapy for localized aggressive lymphoma in elderly patients. A study by the Groupe d' Etude des Lymphomes de l'Adulte. J Clin Oncol 25:787–92, 2007.

27. AK Ng, PM Mauch. Role of radiation therapy in localized aggressive lymphoma. J Clin Oncol 25:757–59, 2007.

28. TP Miller, S Dahlberg, JR Cassady, et al. Chemotherapy alone compared with chemotherapy plus radiotherapy for localized intermediate- and high grade non-Hodgkin's lymphoma. N J Engl Med 339:21–26, 1998.

29. K Ng. Diffuse large B-cell lymphoma. Semin Radiat Oncol 169–75, 2007.

30. F Reyes, E Lepage, G Ganem, et al. Groupe d'Etude des Lymphomes de l'Adulte (GELA). ACVBP versus CHOP plus radiotherapy for localized aggressive lymphoma. N Engl J Med 352:1197–1205, 2005.

31. DO Persky, JM Unger, CM Spier, et al. Phase II study of rituximab plus three cycles of CHOP and involved-field radiotherapy for patients with limited-stage aggressive B-cell lymphoma: Southwest Oncology Group study 0014. J Clin Oncol 26:2258–63, 2008.

32. TN Shenkier, N Voss, R Fairey, et al. Brief chemotherapy and involved-region irradiation for limited-stage diffuse large-cell lymphoma: an 18-year experience from the British Columbia Cancer Agency. J Clin Oncol 20:197–204, 2002.

33. BS Hoppe, CH Moskowitz, DA Filippa, et al. Involved-field radiotherapy before high-dose therapy and autologous stem-cell rescue in diffuse large-cell lymphoma: long-term disease control and toxicity. J Clin Oncol 26:1858–64, 2008.

34. A Aviles, N Neri, S Delgado, et al. Residual disease after chemotherapy in aggressive malignant lymphoma. The role of radiotherapy. Med Oncol 22:383–87, 2005.

35. M Pfreundschuh, L Trumper, Oånsterborg A, et al., for the MabThera International Trial (MInT) Group. CHOP-like chemotherapy plus rituximab versus CHOP-like chemotherapy alone in young patients with good-prognosis diffuse large-B-cell lymphoma: a randomised controlled trial by the MabThera International Trial (MInT) Group. Lancet Oncol 7:379–91, 2006.

36. PL Zinzani, M Tani, S Fanti, et al. A phase II trial of CHOP chemotherapy followed by yttrium 90 ibritumomab tiuxeta (Zevalin) for previously untreated elderly diffuse large B-cell lymphoma patients. Ann Oncol 19:769–73, 2008.

37. AK Ng. Diffuse large B-cell lymphoma. Semin Radiat Oncol 17:169–75, 2007.

APPENDIX A

Table A.1 DLBCL in NHL Pathologic Classification Systems

Rappaport (1966)	Diffuse histiocytic lymphoma
Kiel (1974)	Centroblastic lymphoma
	B-immunoblastic lymphoma
	B-large cell anaplastic lymphoma
Lukes-Collins (1974)	Large cleaved follicular center cell lymphoma
	Large non-cleaved follicular center cell lymphoma
	B-immunoblastic lymphoma
Working Formulation (1982)	Diffuse mixed small and large cell lymphoma (group F)
	Diffuse large cell lymphoma (group G)
	Large cell immunoblastic lymphoma (group H)
REAL (1994); WHO (2001)	Diffuse large B-cell lymphoma

Adapted from Reference 5.

Table A.2 Outcome According to Risk Group Defined by the International Index (All Patients)

Risk of death by group	No. of risk factors	CR rates (%)	5-year RFS (%)	5-year OS (%)
Low	0 or 1	87	70	73
Low-intermediate	2	67	50	51
High-intermediate	3	55	49	43
High	4 or 5	44	40	26

Table A.3 Outcome According to Risk Group Defined by the International Index: Patients $\leq$60 (Referred to as Age-adjusted IPI)

Risk of death by group	No. of risk factors	CR rates (%)	5-year RFS (%)	5-year OS (%)
Low	0	92	86	83
Low-intermediate	1	78	66	69
High-intermediate	2	57	53	46
High	3	46	58	32

Table A.4 Five-year Overall Survival Rates for Patients over 60 Years

Risk of death by group	No. of risk factors	5-year OS (%)
Low	0	56
Low-intermediate	1	44
High-intermediate	2	37
High	3	21

APPENDIX B
Explanation of Determination of International Prognostic Factors

The Ann Arbor staging system (I–IV) was used and stage II was subdivided between II non-bulky (largest tumor dimension <10 cm) and II bulky (largest tumor dimension ≥10 cm). The median size of the bulky disease was 7 cm, range 1–34 cm. In 26% of the patients, the dimension of the largest tumor was unknown before treatment and stage IV contained the most patients. "B" symptoms – recurrent fever (temperature <38.3°C [101°F]), night sweats or loss of more than 10% of body weight – were included in the initial analysis, but not retained as one of the prognostic factors.

The clinical features evaluated included the following factors:

Age

≤ 60 vs. <60

Ann Arbor tumor stage

I
II (tumor <10 cm), II (tumor ≥10 cm), II (tumor size unknown)
III
IV

Serum lactate dehydrogenase concentration

≤1×normal vs. <1×normal

Performance status (PS) based on ECOG criteria: collapsed as ambulatory (0 or 1) (equivalent Karnofsky score ≥80%) versus non-ambulatory (2, 3 or 4) (equivalent Karnofsky score ≤70)

0: Fully active
1: Ambulatory
2: Bedridden <50% time
3: Bedridden ≥50% time
4: Completely bedridden

Number of extranodal sites

None
1 site
<1 site
Unknown

List of risk factors for all patients (14)

Age (≤ 60 vs. <60)
Serum LDH (≤1×normal vs. <1×normal)
Performance status (0 or 1 vs. 2–4)
Stage (I or II vs. III or IV)
Extranodal involvement (≤1 site vs. <1)

Age-adjusted list of risk factors (≤60 years old) (14)

Stage (I or II vs. III or IV)
Serum LDH (≤1×normal vs. <1×normal)
Performance status (0 or 1 vs. 2–4)

50

8 Primary Central Nervous System Lymphomas

Erin S Murphy and Samuel T Chao

Image-guided Radiotherapy and Central Nervous System Lymphoma

Primary central nervous system lymphoma (PCNSL) is a malignant non-Hodgkin's lymphoma (NHL) arising in the central nervous system (CNS) [1]. This disease represents 3–7% of primary brain tumors [1,2]. Treatment strategies vary, but usually involve chemotherapy and whole brain radiation therapy (WBRT). Imaging (computed tomography [CT], magnetic resonance imaging [MRI], single-photon emission computed tomography [SPECT] and positron emission tomography [PET]) can aid in the diagnosis and guide treatment, and may also be useful in assessing a patient's response to therapy and identifying tumor recurrences. Studies that have investigated the role of imaging with PCNSL are small, and newer modalities need further investigation.

Epidemiology

The incidence of PCNSLs is rising in both immunocompetent and immunocompromised individuals [3]. In fact, from 1973 to 1992, frequency increased from 2.5 to 30 cases per 10 million, with most occurring in immunocompromised patients, many secondary to human immunodeficiency virus (HIV) [4]. The incidence of HIV-related primary CNS lymphoma has decreased in the era of highly active antiretroviral therapy [5]. Nonetheless, the overall incidence of PCNSL continues to rise. Immunocompromised patients tend to be younger with the median age at diagnosis of these patients being 31 vs. 55 years in immunocompetent patients [13]. PCNSL arises from the brain parenchyma, eyes, meninges or spinal cord in the absence of systemic disease [6]. Approximately 20–25% of patients with PCNSL also present with intraocular lymphoma [7]. Almost 90% of patients who present with primary intraocular lymphoma will experience cerebral involvement [8,9].

There are two patterns of intraocular lymphoma: lymphoma involving the optic nerve, retina and vitreous, and lymphoma involving the uveal tract [10]. Bilateral involvement is common, although many patients present with symptoms affecting one eye. Primary leptomeningeal lymphoma without parenchymal disease is rare and accounts for only 7% of all cases of PCNSL. Primary spinal cord lymphoma is even less common, accounting for 0.1–6.5% of all lymphomas [11]. In previous reports, the incidence of meningeal seeding from parenchymal PCNSL varied from 5 to 69% [2,12].

Histology

PCNSLs are most commonly aggressive B-cell lymphomas. In immunocompetent patients, PCNSLs present as diffuse large B-cell lymphomas (DLBCL) with similar immunophenotyping to DLBCL outside the CNS [2]. T-cell lymphomas have been reported, but are rare. Patients with HIV present with aggressive or high-grade histopathology; approximately 90% are associated with Epstein-Barr virus (EBV) [2].

Risk Factors

In immunocompromised individuals, EBV infection is a risk factor for PCNSL. The virus most likely transforms chronically activated B cells into malignant lymphoma cells. Experiments have shown that EBV can immortalize B cells in vitro and suggest that the viral latent membrane protein 1 (LMP1) plays a role in the oncogenic process [14]. In rare cases, antecedent demyelinating disease, either sporadic or Lyme disease-related, may correlate with the development of PCNSL [15].

Clinical Presentation

The presenting symptoms relate to the site of involvement: intracranial lesion (solitary or multiple), diffuse leptomeningeal or periventricular lesions, vitreous or uveal deposits and/or intradural spinal cord lesion. Although there are some reports of a neurologic prodrome lasting for years before the diagnosis of PCNSL [2], symptoms usually emerge quickly due to rapid tumor growth. Lethargy, confusion and impaired memory are often the initial signs. Immunocompetent patients more often have specific symptoms, whereas patients with HIV more often have diffuse disease, leading to altered mental status, more generalized signs and seizures [2]. Patients with intraocular lymphoma usually present with blurred vision or floaters in their visual fields.

Patient Evaluation

A complete history is taken with emphasis on the duration of symptoms. Risk factors are assessed, including HIV/AIDS and immunosuppressive therapies. A physical examination addresses all lymph node groups. Older men should undergo a testicular examination. It is also important to evaluate cognitive function by performing a Mini Mental Status Examination (MMSE) or other neurocognitive tests. This will generate baseline data that can be compared with follow-up examinations. An ophthalmologic examination is performed. A slit lamp examination may reveal vitreous opacity or yellowish-white infiltrates at the subretinal pigment epithelial level [16].

Laboratory examinations include HIV testing, lactate dehydrogenase (LDH), complete blood count (CBC) and comprehensive metabolic panel (CMP). A lumbar puncture is performed if there is no evidence of increased cranial pressure. The spinal fluid should undergo analysis for cytology, flow cytometry, EBV polymerase chain reaction (PCR) and immunophenotypic analysis. Cingolani and colleagues evaluated the role of PCR of EBV-DNA from cerebrospinal fluid (CSF) as a diagnostic tool for AIDS-related PCNSL and reported a sensitivity and specificity of PCR for EBV-DNA detection in lumbar CSF of 80% (95% confidence interval [CI] = 60.9–91.6%) and 100% (95% CI = 92.6–100%), respectively [17].

A histopathologic confirmation of the diagnosis is necessary because a presumptive diagnosis based on either MRI appearance or tumor response to steroids may lead to mismanagement of the patient. The differential diagnosis is extensive and includes multiple sclerosis, sarcoidosis and occasional gliomas that may have a similar appearance on imaging, clinical presentation and transient response to corticosteroids [18].

A stereotactic needle biopsy is the first choice to obtain a tissue sample in these patients. Several techniques have been investigated and reported. Large-caliber (12–17 gauge) biopsy instruments have been used, with or without stereotactic guidance, with reported diagnostic success rates between 79 and 95% [19]. Diagnostic needle biopsies have reported morbidity and mortality outcomes of up to 14 and 4.7%, respectively [20].

A group from Tufts University presented their outcomes from 130 fine-needle aspiration CNS biopsies using a 22-gauge needle under CT guidance without stereotactic instrumentation guidance. They reported a success rate of 75%, and had no procedure-related morbidity or mortality [19]. A surgical resection does not improve the clinical outcomes in these patients and is rarely necessary. If there is evidence of ocular or CSF involvement, a vitrectomy, vitreous aspirate or CSF cytology can be used to establish the tissue diagnosis.

Evidence of systemic disease in patients thought to have PCNSL is found in about 4–8% of cases [21,22]. Because of this possibility, the International Primary CNS Lymphoma Collaborative Group recommends a CT of the chest, abdomen and pelvis, and bone marrow biopsy for all patients enrolling in clinical trials [18]. Others recommend this same systemic evaluation for patients who present with B symptoms.

Imaging

In immunocompetent individuals, CT of the head usually reveals a focal lesion that is homogeneously enhancing, often periventricular in location, and involves the corpus callosum, thalamus or basal ganglia. An unenhanced CT often shows an isodense or hyperdense lesion [23]. The lesions have variable appearances on MRI and may also reveal edema and mass effect. A report of 23 patients with PCNSL revealed that all lesions were isointense or hypointense on T1-weighted images and 53% were isointense or hypointense on T2-weighted images (Fig. 8.1a, b). Of the patients who received intravenous (IV) contrast, the lesions were enhanced in 91% (Fig. 8.2a, b). The patients without enhancing lesions had been previously treated with corticosteroids prior to the MRI. This study also reports that immunocompromised patients were more likely to have ring-enhancing lesions [24].

In contrast to immunocompetent individuals, the lesions of immunocompromised patients tend to have more heterogeneous patterns of enhancement. These patients are also more likely to present with multiple lesions [23]. Magnetic resonance spectroscopy reveals masses with diminished concentrations of N-acetylaspartate and elevated ratios (>3:1) of choline to creatine [2]. Calcification, necrosis and cystic appearance are uncommon with PCNSL.

Recent reports show that thallium-201 (^{201}Tl) SPECT may be able to differentiate between cerebral lymphoma and non-neoplastic lesions in patients with AIDS presenting with focal brain lesions [25]. Antinori and colleagues attempted to improve the diagnostic accuracy of ^{201}Tl SPECT by combining the test with EBV DNA. The presence of increased SPECT activity and/or positive EBV DNA gave a sensitivity of 100% and a negative predictive value of 100% [26].

Several small studies have investigated the role of PET in diagnosing PCNSL and assessing treatment response. In particular, one small study reported on the usefulness of PET in AIDS patients with CNS lesions [27]. This group in Germany studied ^{18}F-fluorodeoxyglucose (FDG)-PET scans of 11 AIDS patients with a known diagnosis of CNS lesions. They found that in the patients with cerebral infections, including toxoplasmosis and tuberculosis, the standardized uptake value (SUV) ratio was significantly ($p<0.05$) lower than the SUV ratio in patients with lymphoma (range: 0.3–0.7 vs. 1.7–3.1) [27]. Their findings suggest that FDG-PET may help establish a clinical diagnosis and lead to appropriate therapy in patients with PCNSL.

Duke University reported on a group of 10 patients (one with AIDS) with biopsy-proven PCNSL and compared the FDG-PET results with other malignant brain tumors. The results

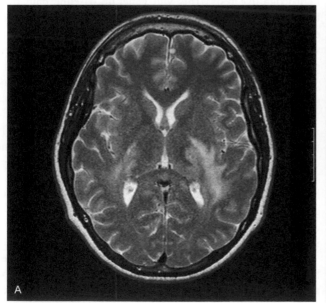
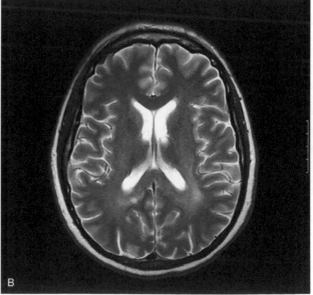

Figure 8.1 (A) T2 MRI of a patient with PCNSL, note the diffuse nature of the disease. (B) T2 MRI of the same patient after treatment with high-dose methotrexate.

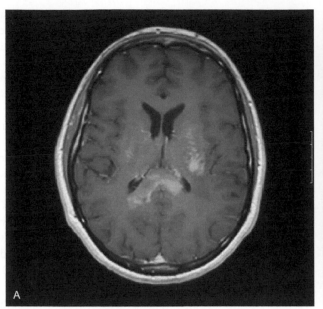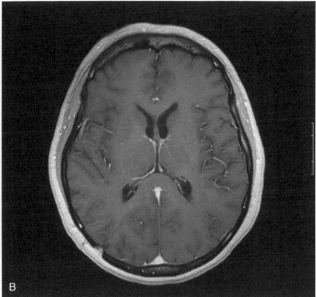

Figure 8.2 (A) T1 post-contrast MRI of a patient with PCNSL, note the cotton-wool appearance of the infiltrating tumor. (B) T1 post-contrast MRI of a patient with PCNSL after treatment with high-dose methotrexate.

demonstrated that the accumulation of FDG in primary CNS lymphoma is similar to that seen in anaplastic gliomas and is significantly more prominent than in low-grade astrocytomas ($p=0.001$). Therefore, although it is difficult to distinguish PCNSL from high-grade gliomas, it is likely that the level of FDG uptake can separate PCNSL from low-grade gliomas. The difference in FDG uptake between steroid-treated and untreated cases of primary CNS lymphoma did not reach statistical significance ($p=0.40$), most likely because of the small sample size [28].

The Mayo Clinic performed a retrospective review of the diagnostic role of PET/CT in 25 HIV-negative PCNSL patients. Their report showed a variable sensitivity depending on the site of the PCNSL: 87% in the brain, 80% in the spine/nerves and only 20% in the eyes [29]. Case reports have shown that PET/CT may be useful at detecting occult systemic disease not seen on CT alone, but this is not the standard of care [21].

Ogawa and colleagues performed a study in which patients with histologically verified PCNSL were imaged with PET using carbon-11 methionine, CT and MRI before and after radiotherapy. They demonstrated that PCNSL had an increased uptake of the C-11 methionine. Interestingly, the area of increased C-11 methionine uptake was most often larger than the enhancing lesions seen on CT or MRI. However, this difference in size may be related to the different mechanism of tracer uptake for the respective imaging modality. The paper stated that for MRI and CT, the contrast enhancement occurs because the blood-brain barrier has been disrupted, whereas the increased accumulation of C-11 methionine occurs via carrier-mediated active transport by the tumor. These differences may account for the larger area of C-11 methionine uptake and the fact that decreased uptake after radiation correlates with cell death and or inactivity. For the patients who had repeat PET with C-11 methionine within 1 month of completion of radiation therapy (RT), the extent and degree of C-11 methionine was markedly reduced [30]. Therefore, C-11 methionine PET may be a useful tool for diagnosing

and assessing the therapeutic response of radiation in these patients.

More recently, a group in Japan investigated several parameters of FDG-PET in immunocompetent PCNSL patients before and after treatment. The investigators used dynamic image acquisition to model regional FDG transport and determine phosphorylation rates to establish the kinetic parameters of the tumor. They found that the kinetic variables and cerebral metabolic rate of glucose were significantly higher in the tumor than in normal grey matter. Because it assesses the consumption of glucose, FDG-PET is a useful tool for determining the metabolic activity of a lesion and may correlate with the degree of malignancy of the tumor. Also, the pre-treatment kinetics and metabolic rate of glucose were significantly higher than the post-treatment values, suggesting these values are a useful means of evaluating response to therapy [31].

Prognostic Factors

In 2003, the International Extranodal Lymphoma Study Group (IELSG) published a consensus prognostic scoring system that included five risk factors for poor performance: age >60, Eastern Cooperative Oncology Group performance status >1, elevated serum LDH level, elevated CSF protein, and involvement of deep regions of the brain (periventricular areas, corpus callosum, basal ganglia, brainstem and cerebellum) [32]. More recently, the Memorial Sloan-Kettering Cancer Center (MSKCC) presented a recursive partitioning analysis (RPA) classification of 282 patients from their institution with three distinct prognostic classes: class 1 (patients <50 years), class 2 (patients ≥50; Karnofsky performance score [KPS] ≥70) and class 3 (patients ≥50; KPS <70). This system correlates with overall and failure-free survival and was validated with data from three prospective Radiation Therapy Oncology Group (RTOG) trials [33]. Of note, age is the most important prognostic factor. The RPA class 1 patients had a median survival of 8.5 years, whereas the median survival for classes 2 and 3 was 3.2 and 1.1 year, respectively.

Treatment

Historically, PCNSL was treated with WBRT alone with doses of 40–60 Gy. Although these tumors are quite radiosensitive, the rates of recurrence were high and overall survival was poor. In the early 1980s, RTOG conducted a phase II trial of 41 patients with PCNSL treated with whole brain irradiation to 40 Gy and a 20-Gy boost to the tumor plus a 2-cm margin. The overall median survival was 11.6 months with 48% of patients surviving 1 year and 28% surviving 2 years. Patients younger than 60 years had a median survival of 23.1 months, while those who were 60 years of age and older had a median survival of 7.6 months [34]. (See Table 8.1 for summary of trials.)

In an effort to improve survival, researchers eventually added chemotherapy to the treatment plan. The addition of chemotherapy proved to increase survival compared to radiation alone. In general, multi-agent chemotherapy regimens are more effective than single agents in the setting of aggressive systemic lymphomas. Therefore, multi-agent regimens were incorporated into therapy regimens for PCNSL.

Patient survival improved considerably in several phase II studies that used upfront methotrexate (MTX) combined with WBRT [35,36]. In 1985, the MSKCC was one of the first groups to investigate the addition of chemotherapy to WBRT. They enrolled 31 newly diagnosed PCNSL patients on a protocol that consisted of IV (1 g/m²) and intra-Ommaya MTX followed by WBRT 40 Gy plus a boost of 14.4 Gy followed by two cycles of high-dose cytarabine (Ara-C; 3 g/m²). During the same period, 16 patients were treated with RT alone, either because they refused chemotherapy or had already initiated the radiation. The 31 patients who received the MTX-based chemotherapy in addition to radiation

had a median survival rate of 42.5 months, which was substantially better than the 21.7 months of those who had received radiation alone [37]. The difference in survival was not statistically significant, but there was a significant difference in time to relapse in favor of the chemotherapy group [37]. In an update, Abrey et al. reported a median cause-specific survival of 42 months for the patients receiving IV and intrathecal MTX followed by WBRT and Ara-C [35]. Of note, 10 of the 31 patients in this trial had delayed neurotoxicity.

In 1988, the RTOG opened a study to investigate a different chemotherapy regimen, utilizing the same agents that were successful in systemic NHL. Their phase I/II study assessed upfront cyclophosphamide, doxorubicin, vincristine and dexamethasone (CHOD) chemotherapy followed by WBRT to 41.4 Gy and a tumor boost of 18 Gy, all given in 1.8 Gy per fraction. After two cycles of CHOD, the patients were reassessed with a head CT. If there was no evidence of progression, then the patients received a third cycle of CHOD prior to WBRT. If the patients showed progression, they went directly to WBRT. All of the patients had CSF analysis for cytology. If the patients had positive CSF cytology, then they also received intrathecal MTX. Unfortunately, the median survival of 16.1 months was not significantly longer than the median survival associated with radiation alone seen in RTOG 8315 [38]. Patient age <60 years was found to be a significant prognostic factor with respect to survival on univariate analysis. During chemotherapy, about 80% of patients experienced grade 3 or 4 hematologic toxicity. During RT, all but two patients reported grade 1 or 2 toxicity [38].

In an effort to further improve survival from their initial experience, the MSKCC treatment protocol was adapted to include upfront procarbazine and vincristine. Procarbazine had proven

Table 8.1 Summary of Studies Investigating Treatment Strategies for Primary CNS Lymphoma

Study	No of patients	Chemotherapy	Radiation therapy	Median survival
RTOG 8315 Nelson et al. (1992)[34]	41	None	WBRT 40 Gy +20 Gy boost to GTV +2 cm	12.2 months (KPS 70–100: 21.1 months, KPS 40–60: 5.6 months, <60 years: 23.1 months, >60 years: 7.6 months)
DeAngelis et al. (1992)[37]	31	Group A: IV (1 g/m²) and IT MTX+adjuvant cytarabine	WBRT 40 Gy +14.4 Gy boost to tumor bed	Group A: 42.5 months
	16	Group B: none		Group B: 21.7 months
RTOG 8806 Schultz et al. (1996)[38]	52	CHOD (cyclophosphamide, doxorubicin, vincristine and dexamethasone)	WBRT 41.4 Gy +18 Gy boost to CTV +2 cm	16.1 months
Abrey et al. (2000)[39]	52	MPV (methotrexate (3.5 g/m²), procarbazine, vincristine)+IT MTX ± adjuvant cytarabine	30 patients received WBRT 45 Gy/22 patients deferred RT	60 months
RTOG 9310 DeAngelis et al. (2002)[36]	102	MPV (methotrexate (2.5 g/m²), procarbazine, vincristine)+IT MTX + adjuvant cytarabine	WBRT 45 Gy (changed to 36 Gy in 1.2 Gy BID for the last 16 patients)	36.9 months (<60 years: 50.4 months, >60 years: 21.8 months)
Pels et al. (2003)[44]	65	MTX (5 g/m²), cytarabine, dexamethasone, vincristine, ifosfamide, cyclophosphamide+IT MTX, prednisolone and cytarabine	None	50 months (age <61 years, MS: not reached, age >60, MS: 34 months
NABTT 9607 Batchelor et al. (2003)[43]	25	MTX (8 g/m²) every 14 days until CR or 8 cycles	None	22.8+ months (not yet reached)
McAllister et al. (2000)[4]	74	BBBD-IA MTX (2.5 g), etoposide +/or cyclophosphamide, ± procarbazine	None	40.7 months

benefit against NHL and could penetrate the blood-brain barrier. Vincristine was also useful for NHL, and it was thought that it could be effective in the brain in areas of decreased integrity of the blood-brain barrier. Therefore, the new regimen consisted of IV MTX (3.5 g/m²), procarbazine (100 mg/m²/d), vincristine (1.4 mg/m²), intra-Ommaya MTX (12 mg) and adjuvant Ara-C. Of 52 patients who received this regimen, 30 received 45-Gy WBRT and 22 deferred the WBRT. Patients who were older than 60 years were offered radiation deferment. The objective MRI response rate was 90%. The reported overall median survival was 60 months. Interestingly, the median survival for the older patients who deferred initial radiation treatment was 33 months compared with 32 months for those who received it upfront. Of note, patients older than 60 years who underwent radiation had a significantly higher rate of delayed neurotoxicity of 83% compared with 6% in the younger population. The symptoms of neurotoxicity included memory loss, behavioral disturbance, urinary incontinence, falls and unsteady gait [39].

Because the addition of procarbazine and vincristine to MTX and WBRT proved to prolong survival, this regimen was utilized for a prospective multi-institutional trial. RTOG 9310/Southwest Oncology Group (SWOG) conducted a trial in which immunocompetent PCNSL patients received IV MTX, vincristine, procarbazine and intraventricular MTX followed by WBRT and high-dose Ara-C. The agents were given in a similar manner to the MSKCC regimen, but the MTX was reduced from 3.5 to 2.5 g/m² because of the concern for possible acute MTX-related toxicity. The dose of whole brain radiation was 45 Gy given in 1.8 Gy per fraction. Midway through the study, in an attempt to decrease neurotoxicity, patients who obtained a complete response to chemotherapy were given 36-Gy WBRT in 1.2 Gy twice a day fractions for 15 fractions. In this study, the median survival was 50.4 months in patients younger than 60 years and 21.8 months in those aged 60 and older. There was no difference in progression-free survival or overall survival for the different WBRT regimens in the patients who achieved a complete response to chemotherapy [36]. The severe delayed neurotoxicity rate in this trial was 15% (12 of 82 patients who received WBRT) and included eight deaths. The severe delayed neurotoxicity was primarily characterized as leukoencephalopathy and presented at a median time of 504 days after the initiation of WBRT. The rates of leukoencephalopathy were equally distributed among patients younger than 60 years and those aged 60 years and older [36]. Because of these high rates of neurotoxicity, particularly for patients older than 60 years, as seen in previous studies, there has been a trend to defer WBRT for relapsed disease.

Bessell et al. attempted to reduce the dose of WBRT in hopes of reducing neurotoxicity. They reported two consecutive trials. In both trials, treatment consisted of CHOD/carmustine, vincristine, Ara-C and methotrexate (BVAM) chemotherapy followed by WBRT. The first trial delivered 45-Gy WBRT to all patients and the second trial delivered 45 Gy to patients with a partial response to chemotherapy and 30.6 Gy to patients with a complete response. The recurrence rate was 29% from the first trial and 70% in the second trial with the response-adapted RT. In particular, for patients less than 60 years of age, the 3-year risk of relapse was 25 vs. 83%, respectively. For patients younger than 60 years of age, the 3-year overall survival was decreased from 92 to 60% for those who

received 45 vs. 30.6 Gy, respectively. Therefore, the recommendation was to not decrease the WBRT dose for patients less than 60 years old who achieve a complete response to chemotherapy [40]. However, the subset analysis from RTOG 9310 has shown survival to be comparable between patients receiving chemotherapy followed by WBRT delivered with 36 Gy in 1.2 Gy twice daily fractions and those receiving chemotherapy followed by 45-Gy WBRT. Of the patients who were evaluated with a MMSE, there was no difference at 8 months between the two groups. Two of the 16 patients (13%) in the hyperfractionated (HFX) group and 6 of 66 patients (9%) in the 45-Gy group developed grade 5 (fatal) neurotoxicity. However, none of the HFX group had grade 5 neurotoxicity at 2 years compared to 5% of the 45-Gy group. Therefore, the HFX regimen delayed severe neurotoxicity, but did not reduce the rate of neurotoxicity [41]. Because of the conflicting data, it remains unclear if RT dose reduction improves safety [6].

Nonetheless, there have been multiple investigations that delay the WBRT and use WBRT as salvage for failure of primary chemotherapy. Several trials for newly diagnosed PCNSL have omitted upfront radiation and have shown comparable median survival to treatment with MTX and WBRT [42–44]. The New Approaches to Brain Tumor Therapy (NABTT) CNS Consortium conducted a trial that consisted of 25 patients with PCNSL who received high-dose IV MTX (8 g/m²) q 2 weeks until a complete response or for a total of eight cycles; the RT was deferred until relapse. Radiographic response was the primary endpoint, and the results showed a response rate of 74%, but only 52% had a complete response. The median survival had not yet been reached at more than 22.8 months of follow-up. Of note, the patients were followed with a MMSE to assess neurotoxicity. Of the 19 patients with at least one follow-up MMSE score, only one decreased from baseline (from a score of 29 to 27) [43].

McAllister and colleagues report on a series of 74 patients with PCNSL who received blood-brain barrier disruption (BBBD)-enhanced chemotherapy and omitted RT. The patients were treated with intra-arterial cyclophosphamide and MTX (2.5 g/m² per cycle) after osmotic BBBD and etoposide and/or procarbazine. The median survival was 40.7 months. Overall, 48 patients (65%) had an objective complete response and 36 patients continued to exhibit complete responses after 1 year of BBBD-enhanced chemotherapy. None of the 36 patients with a sustained response had a decline of cognition evaluated by neuropsychological tests or clinical examinations [42].

Similarly, a group in Germany reported on a series of 65 patients treated with MTX (5 g/m²), cytarabine, dexamethasone, vincristine, ifosfamide, cyclophosphamide and intraventricular MTX, prednisolone and cytarabine, with deferred radiation. The response was based on MRI: 61% achieved a complete response, 10% achieved a partial response and 19% progressed during therapy. The median time to failure was 21 months, and the median survival was 50 months. In 30 patients younger than 61 years, neither the median survival nor median time to failure had been reached at the time of publication [44].

Salvage Treatment

At Massachusetts General Hospital, 27 patients who failed to respond to high-dose MTX therapy were treated with salvage WBRT with a median dose of 36 Gy. There was a radiographic response rate of 74% with a 37% complete response rate and a 37% partial response rate. The median survival for these patients was 10.9 months. The analysis from this study found that age (<60 years) and response to WBRT were predictors for survival. They reported a 15% rate of late neurotoxicity, which correlated with a total dose >36 Gy. No patients who received a fractional daily dose of <1.8 Gy experienced late neurotoxicity [45].

High-dose MTX has also been used for salvage therapy. Plotkin and colleagues report a study of 22 patients with relapsed PCNSL who either had a complete response to initial MTX-based chemotherapy or received MTX after gross total resection or interstitial radiation. Two of the 22 patients had surgical resections before chemotherapy, 5 received focal radiation before chemotherapy and 3 received other chemotherapeutic agents besides MTX. At relapse, all patients were re-treated with high-dose MTX. Nineteen patients received cycles of HD-MTX at 8 g/m^2, two patients at 3.5 g/m^2 and one patient at 3 g/m^2. The overall response rates were 91% to first salvage (20 of 22 patients) and 100% to second salvage (4 of 4 patients), with a median survival of 61.9 months after first relapse [46].

A few small studies have investigated high-dose myeloablative chemotherapy followed by autologous stem cell transplant (ASCT) for relapsed disease or for upfront treatment in patients with poor prognostic factors. Brevet and colleagues reported a series of six patients treated with induction chemotherapy followed by intensive chemotherapy and ASCT. Four of the six patients had a durable response with a median survival of 35.5 months. Two patients died from relapse at 19 and 23 months [47]. Another trial from Germany included 30 PCNSL patients <65 years old. The goal of therapy was to improve survival and decrease toxicity. The treatment consisted of three cycles of MTX (8 g/m^2), cytarabine (3 g/m^2) and thiotepa (40 mg/m^2) followed by stem-cell harvest and carmustine (400 mg/m^2) and thiotepa (two doses of 5 mg/kg body weight), followed by ASCT. Then, WBRT was given to a dose of 45 Gy in twice daily fractions of 1 Gy per fraction. Overall, the therapy was well tolerated with a 5-year overall survival probability of 69% for all patients and 87% for the patients who received the ASCT [48].

Future Directions

An active phase IV randomized trial in Germany (G-PCNSL-SG1) is investigating the effects of six 14-week cycles of high-dose MTX (4 g/m^2 IV) followed by immediate WBRT versus WBRT given at relapse of disease. The dose of WBRT will be 45 Gy in 1.5 Gy per fraction given over 6 weeks, and the primary endpoints are progression free and overall survival. If the patients' disease fails to respond to the initial MTX therapy, they will be further randomized to WBRT or high-dose Ara-C. This study will hopefully provide information regarding the appropriate timing of WBRT and investigate the efficacy of high-dose Ara-C as a single second-line treatment.

The RTOG is enrolling patients on RTOG-0227, a phase I/II study investigating the combination of MTX, rituximab and temozolomide followed by RT and adjuvant temozolomide for patients with PCNSL. They added temozolomide to the regimen because it can cross the blood-brain barrier and rituximab because it directly targets B lymphocytes. Although this drug does not readily cross the blood-brain barrier, it is thought that with an

enhancing tumor, at least part of the barrier is non-functioning. The radiation dose will be 36 Gy given in twice daily fractions in an attempt to decrease long-term neurotoxicity. Temozolomide will be continued at a dose of 200 mg/m^2 per day for 5 days every 4 weeks for a total of 10 cycles after RT with the goal of decreasing tumor recurrence.

Several other institutions have open studies investigating various chemotherapy combinations for patients with newly diagnosed PCNSL. The goal is to get more drugs across the blood-brain barrier to enhance the treatment for this disease. The Oregon Health and Science University has an open trial (OHSU-1012) investigating the combination of rituximab in combination with carboplatin, BBBD with mannitol, and delayed sodium thiosulfate in patients with newly diagnosed PCNSL. Again, with the goal of enhancing chemotherapy regimens and deferring WBRT, the Cancer and Leukemia Group B has an open phase II trial (CALGB 50202) for newly diagnosed PCNSL. With a similar strategy to the open RTOG study, they have incorporated temozolomide and rituximab in their regimen. In this study, the patients will receive high-dose MTX, leukovorin, temozolamide and rituximab, followed by cytarabine and etoposide. There are also several phase II trials investigating different chemotherapy regimens for refractory or relapsed PCNSL.

Conclusion

Over the last 30 years, there has been an improvement in the treatment strategies for PCNSL. These improvements have prolonged survival in this patient population. However, the high rates of local recurrence suggest room for continued improvement. At this time, there is little role for image-guided RT in the management of PCNSL. The diffuse nature of this disease requires radiation treatment of the whole brain and meninges. Currently, imaging can guide both the diagnosis and treatment plan for these patients. Imaging may also be a useful tool in assessing response to therapy and to determine possible recurrences. The studies that investigate the role of imaging with PCNSL are small, but show a potential benefit to the overall treatment plan for these patients. Hopefully, with improved chemotherapeutic regimens and better imaging, image-guided RT may be feasible. This would reduce neurotoxicity, which is the most concerning complication of radiation when added to chemotherapy. Image-guided RT may one day be used to target residual disease identified on imaging following chemotherapy.

REFERENCES

1. GD Shah, LM DeAngelis. Treatment of primary central nervous system lymphoma. Hematol/Oncol Clin North Am 19(4):611–27, v, 2005.
2. FH Hochberg, JM Baehring, EP Hochberg. CNS Primary lymphoma. Nat Clin Pract 3(1): 24–35, 2007.
3. LM Deangelis. Current management of primary central nervous system lymphoma. Oncology (Williston Park, NY) 9(1):63–71; discussion 5–6, 8, 1995.
4. BW Corn, SM Marcus, A Topham, et al. Will primary central nervous system lymphoma be the most frequent brain tumor diagnosed in the year 2000? Cancer 79(12):2409–13, 1997.
5. E Gerstner, T Batchelor. Primary CNS lymphoma. Expert Rev Anticancer Ther 7(5):689–700, 2007.

6. LM Deangelis, FM Iwamoto. An update on therapy of primary central nervous system lymphoma. Hematology/ Education Program of the American Society of Hematology. Am Soc Hematol 311–16, 2006.

7. N Tuaillon, CC Chan. Molecular analysis of primary central nervous system and primary intraocular lymphomas. Curr Mol Med 1(2):259–72, 2001.

8. DH Char, BM Ljung, T Miller, et al. Primary intraocular lymphoma (ocular reticulum cell sarcoma) diagnosis and management. Ophthalmology 95(5):625–30, 1988.

9. EJ Rockwood, ZN Zakov, JW Bay. Combined malignant lymphoma of the eye and CNS (reticulum-cell sarcoma). Report of three cases. J Neurosurg 61(2):369–74, 1984.

10. SJ Qualman, G Mendelsohn, RB Mann, et al. Intraocular lymphomas. Natural history based on a clinicopathologic study of eight cases and review of the literature. Cancer 52(5):878–86, 1983.

11. M Salvati, L Cervoni, M Artico, et al. Primary spinal epidural non-Hodgkin's lymphomas: a clinical study. Surg Neurol 46(4):339–43; 1996, discussion 43–44.

12. LM DeAngelis, J Yahalom, MH Heinemann, et al. Primary CNS lymphoma: combined treatment with chemotherapy and radiotherapy. Neurology 40(1):80–86, 1990.

13. HA Fine, RJ Mayer. Primary central nervous system lymphoma. Ann Intern Med 119(11):1093–104, 1993.

14. E Cesarman. Epstein-Barr virus (EBV) and lymphomagenesis. Front Biosci 7:e58–65, 2002.

15. K Brecher, FH Hochberg, DN Louis, et al. Case report of unusual leukoencephalopathy preceding primary CNS lymphoma. J Neurol Neurosurg Psychiatry 65(6):917–20, 1998.

16. T Matsuo, A Yamaoka, F Shiraga, et al. Two types of initial ocular manifestations in intraocular-central nervous system lymphoma. Retina (Philadelphia, PA) 18(4):301–7, 1998.

17. A Cingolani, A De Luca, LM Larocca, et al. Minimally invasive diagnosis of acquired immunodeficiency syndrome-related primary central nervous system lymphoma. J Nat Cancer Inst 90(5):364–69, 1998.

18. LE Abrey, TT Batchelor, AJ Ferreri, et al. Report of an international workshop to standardize baseline evaluation and response criteria for primary CNS lymphoma. J Clin Oncol 23(22):5034–43, 2005.

19. RM Seliem, MW Assaad, SJ Gorombey, et al. Fine-needle aspiration biopsy of the central nervous system performed freehand under computed tomography guidance without stereotactic instrumentation. Cancer 99(5):277–84, 2003.

20. S Goldstein, MK Gumerlock, EA Neuwelt. Comparison of CT-guided and stereotaxic cranial diagnostic needle biopsies. J Neurosurg 67(3):341–48, 1987.

21. D Karantanis, BP O'Neill, RM Subramaniam, et al. Contribution of F-18 FDG PET-CT in the detection of systemic spread of primary central nervous system lymphoma. Clin Nucl Med 32(4):271–74, 2007.

22. AJ Ferreri, M Reni, MC Zoldan, et al. Importance of complete staging in non-Hodgkin's lymphoma presenting as a cerebral mass lesion. Cancer 77(5):827–33, 1996.

23. N Erdag, RM Bhorade, RA Alberico, et al. Primary lymphoma of the central nervous system: typical and atypical CT and MR imaging appearances. AJR 176(5):1319–26, 2001.

24. BA Johnson, EK Fram, PC Johnson, et al. The variable MR appearance of primary lymphoma of the central nervous system: comparison with histopathologic features. AJNR 18(3): 563–72, 1997.

25. JP O'Malley, HA Ziessman, PN Kumar, et al. Diagnosis of intracranial lymphoma in patients with AIDS: value of 201TI single-photon emission computed tomography. AJR 163(2): 417–21, 1994.

26. A Antinori, G De Rossi, A Ammassari, et al. Value of combined approach with thallium-201 single-photon emission computed tomography and Epstein-Barr virus DNA polymerase chain reaction in CSF for the diagnosis of AIDS-related primary CNS lymphoma. J Clin Oncol 17(2): 554–60, 1999.

27. K Villringer, H Jager, M Dichgans, et al. Differential diagnosis of CNS lesions in AIDS patients by FDG-PET. J Comput Assist Tomogr 19(4): 532–36, 1995.

28. SS Rosenfeld, JM Hoffman, RE Coleman, et al. Studies of primary central nervous system lymphoma with fluorine-18-fluorodeoxyglucose positron emission tomography. J Nucl Med 33(4): 532–36, 1992.

29. D Karantanis, BP O'Neill, RM Subramaniam, et al. 18F-FDG PET/CT in primary central nervous system lymphoma in HIV-negative patients. Nucl Med Commun 28(11): 834–41, 2007.

30. T Ogawa, I Kanno, J Hatazawa, et al. Methionine PET for follow-up of radiation therapy of primary lymphoma of the brain. Radiographics 14(1): 101–10, 1994.

31. Y Nishiyama, Y Yamamoto, T Monden, et al. Diagnostic value of kinetic analysis using dynamic FDG PET in immunocompetent patients with primary CNS lymphoma. Eur J Nucl Med Mol Imaging 34(1): 78–86, 2007.

32. AJ Ferreri, LE Abrey, JY Blay, et al. Summary statement on primary central nervous system lymphomas from the Eighth International Conference on Malignant Lymphoma, Lugano, Switzerland, June 12 to 15, 2002. J Clin Oncol 21(12): 2407–14, 2003.

33. LE Abrey, L Ben-Porat, KS Panageas, et al. Primary central nervous system lymphoma: the Memorial Sloan-Kettering Cancer Center prognostic model. J Clin Oncol 24(36): 5711–15, 2006.

34. DF Nelson, KL Martz, H Bonner, et al. Non-Hodgkin's lymphoma of the brain: can high dose, large volume radiation therapy improve survival? Report on a prospective trial by the Radiation Therapy Oncology Group (RTOG): RTOG 8315. Int J Radiat Oncol Biol Phys 23(1): 9–17, 1992.

35. LE Abrey, LM DeAngelis, J Yahalom. Long-term survival in primary CNS lymphoma. J Clin Oncol 16(3): 859–63, 1998.

36. LM DeAngelis, W Seiferheld, SC Schold, et al. Combination chemotherapy and radiotherapy for primary central nervous system lymphoma: Radiation Therapy Oncology Group Study 93-10. J Clin Oncol 20(24): 4643–48, 2002.

37. LM DeAngelis, J Yahalom, HT Thaler, et al. Combined modality therapy for primary CNS lymphoma. J Clin Oncol 10(4): 635–43, 1992.

38. C Schultz, C Scott, W Sherman, et al. Preirradiation chemotherapy with cyclophosphamide, doxorubicin, vincristine, and dexamethasone for primary CNS lymphomas: initial

report of Radiation Therapy Oncology Group protocol 88-06. J Clin Oncol 14(2):556–64, 1996.

39. LE Abrey, J Yahalom, LM DeAngelis. Treatment for primary CNS lymphoma: the next step. J Clin Oncol 18(17):3144–50, 2000.

40. EM Bessell, A Lopez-Guillermo, S Villa, et al. Importance of radiotherapy in the outcome of patients with primary CNS lymphoma: an analysis of the CHOD/BVAM regimen followed by two different radiotherapy treatments. J Clin Oncol 20(1):231–36, 2002.

41. B Fisher, W Seiferheld, C Schultz, et al. Secondary analysis of Radiation Therapy Oncology Group study (RTOG) 9310: an intergroup phase II combined modality treatment of primary central nervous system lymphoma. J Neuro-oncol 74(2):201–5, 2005.

42. LD McAllister, ND Doolittle, PE Guastadisegni, et al. Cognitive outcomes and long-term follow-up results after enhanced chemotherapy delivery for primary central nervous system lymphoma. Neurosurgery 46(1):51–60; 2000, discussion 60–61.

43. T Batchelor, K Carson, A O'Neill, et al. Treatment of primary CNS lymphoma with methotrexate and deferred radiotherapy: a report of NABTT 96-07. J Clin Oncol 21(6): 1044–49, 2003.

44. H Pels, IG Schmidt-Wolf, A Glasmacher, et al. Primary central nervous system lymphoma: results of a pilot and phase II study of systemic and intraventricular chemotherapy with deferred radiotherapy. J Clin Oncol 21(24):4489–95, 2003.

45. PL Nguyen, A Chakravarti, DM Finkelstein, et al. Results of whole-brain radiation as salvage of methotrexate failure for immunocompetent patients with primary CNS lymphoma. J Clin Oncol 23(7):1507–13, 2005.

46. SR Plotkin, RA Betensky, FH Hochberg, et al. Treatment of relapsed central nervous system lymphoma with high-dose methotrexate. Clin Cancer Res 10(17):5643–46, 2004.

47. M Brevet, R Garidi, B Gruson, et al. First-line autologous stem cell transplantation in primary CNS lymphoma. J Eur Haematol 75(4):288–92, 2005.

48. G Illerhaus, R Marks, G Ihorst, et al. High-dose chemotherapy with autologous stem-cell transplantation and hyperfractionated radiotherapy as first-line treatment of primary CNS lymphoma. J Clin Oncol 24(24):3865–70, 2006.

9   Orbital B-Cell Lymphoma

Kevin Stephans, Nidhi Sharma, Mohammad Khan and Roger M Macklis

Introduction and Background

Ocular adnexal lymphoma (OAL) represents approximately 10% of orbital neoplasms [1], and 8% of extranodal non-Hodgkin's lymphomas (NHL) [2]. An overall rise in the incidence of orbital lymphomas has been observed in the past few years [3], which may be due to aging of the population, improvements in diagnostic pathology and changes in classification. The incidence of OAL rises with age and it may represent up to 24% of orbital malignancy in this population [4]. Potentially involved primary sites of disease include the orbit, lacrimal gland, eyelids and conjunctiva. Secondary spread to ocular adnexal sites from systemic NHL may also occur.

The most common primary OAL is the low-grade malignant extranodal marginal zone B-cell lymphoma of the mucosa-associated lymphoid tissue (MALT), with almost 100% incidence in conjunctival lesions [5]. Follicular and other low-grade lymphomas are also common, with intermediate- and high-grade lesions seen slightly less often. Issacson and Wright first described MALT lymphomas in 1983, which were adopted as a distinct entity from other low-grade lymphomas in the Revised European-American Classification (REAL) in 1994. This introduces variability in older series of OAL as illustrated by a review of 40 localized orbital lymphomas treated at Stanford from 1977 to 1999. Thirty-one MALT lymphomas were identified, however only 12 of these patients (39%) were initially classified as having MALT histology [6].

Presentation

Patients usually present with mass lesions in the lids or conjunctivae, described as "salmon pink" in color. Retrobulbar tumors may present with swelling and proptosis (with minimal or no pain and inflammation), and associated functional disturbances of extraocular muscles. They occasionally cause foreign body sensation, dry eye or ptosis, which are common symptoms in an older population and have a tendency to be overlooked. These tumors tend to mold themselves around existing orbital structures instead of invading them. Hence, visual loss and diplopia are rare findings, even among larger sized lesions [7]. A total of 10–20% of patients present with bilateral disease. Patients may also present with complaints of the naso-lacrimal system, including epiphora, local swelling and dacryocystitis. In lacrimal sac lymphomas, MALT and diffuse large B-cell lymphomas (DLBCL) occur with roughly equal incidence [8]. The reported frequency of involvement for common sites is displayed in Table 9.1 [9,10].

The propensity for OAL to have systemic involvement at presentation or as a site of failure has been debated. Older series rarely described systemic spread, while more modern estimates provide for systemic disease in as many as one-third of MALT lymphomas [9,11,12] (in contrast to gastric MALT where disseminated disease is relatively rare) and as many as half of all patients with OAL [13–16] over the course of their lifetimes. The differing numbers reported may be due to the small size of the clinical series or to the wide variety of diseases included under this umbrella.

Diagnosis

Conjunctival OALs are diagnosed during routine slit lamp examination in the upper or lower fornix. Clinical appearance does not allow clear distinction between benign and malignant lymphoproliferative lesions. In the eyelid, lacrimal gland and orbit, the lymphoma usually presents as an unseen mass, firm in consistency if palpable, and with variable mobility depending on attachment to surrounding structures. Exophthalmos and decreased retropulsion of the globe are important clinical signs.

On biopsy, the lesion appears as a whitish-pink mass, reflecting leukocytic and vascular characteristics. Histopathology helps confirm the diagnosis, but is not always acquired, particularly for superficial lesions confined to the conjunctiva that are overwhelmingly of MALT histology. Other specific studies include lymphocyte immunophenotypical analysis and molecular genetic studies to identify gene arrangements that indicate clonality and/or translocations. The t(11;18)(q21;q21) translocation, which is associated with antibiotic resistance in gastric MALT, has not been characterized in orbital MALT. However, other imbalances have been identified [17] and are under further investigation, with one group suggesting CD43 expression as a potential unfavorable prognostic factor [18].

Staging includes history and physical examination with attention to B symptoms, complete blood count, erythrocyte sedimentation rate, liver function tests, lactate dehydrogenase, bone marrow biopsy, computed tomography (CT) of the chest, abdomen and pelvis, and immunophenotype analysis. Contrast-enhanced CT or magnetic resonance imaging (MRI) scans of the orbit may be performed to precisely delineate the anatomic extent of the tumor for radiotherapy planning purposes. Conventional imaging does not correlate perfectly with clinical examination and may not always demonstrate lesions. However, it may demonstrate clinically unsuspected retrobulbar involvement in a subset of patients. Positron emission tomography (PET) is increasingly used, particularly as a tool for systemic staging (see below).

Imaging Features of Ocular Adnexal Lymphoma (Computer Tomography and Magnetic Resonance Imaging)

On CT imaging, OALs are typically well-circumscribed, homogenous to slightly streaky-appearing masses, with a density greater than that of surrounding brain tissue. The classic pattern of spread described in early reports is for the lesion to mold to surrounding structures, such as the globe, extraocular muscles, lacrimal gland or bony orbit [19,20]. However, in a more recent study of 87 cases referred to a tertiary center, one-quarter of cases demonstrated invasion into surrounding tissues [21] (bony invasion was rarely seen in <10% of cases). Tissue invasion was significantly more likely in aggressive histologies, but also occasionally seen in

Table 9.1 Subsites of Ocular Adnexal Lymphoma

Site	Incidence (%)
Conjunctiva	20–33
Orbit (lacrimal gland, extraocular muscles, orbital space)	46–74
Eyelid	5–20
Multiple adnexal	10–20

low-grade disease. Most lesions were well circumscribed with density greater than brain tissue, typically only with moderate or minimal contrast enhancement. Calcification was quite rare (6%).

MRI has been slightly more controversial in that some studies have reported hyper-intensity on T2-weighted imaging [22], while others report this to be more variable [21,23]. Moderate enhancement of the lesion with Gadolinium is helpful in defining the extent, although enhancement of the extraocular muscles is often quite similar and may obscure the interface. MRI is probably most useful in cases questioning extension into the central nervous system, sinuses or other adjacent structures. CT is the preferred modality for demonstrating bony erosion.

Positron Emission Tomography in Staging and Definition of Orbital Disease

Studies evaluating ^{18}F-fluorodeoxyglucose (FDG)-PET for staging of OAL have typically demonstrated excellent sensitivity for distant disease, albeit with highly variable sensitivity in defining orbital disease. PET appears to be more sensitive in the detection of systemic disease than conventional imaging in the setting of OAL. This is illustrated by an Australian series examining 11 patients with OAL who also had upfront PET demonstrating increased PET uptake in 5 of 6 patients with systemic spread representing an 83% sensitivity and led to upstaging and change in treatment in 4 patients [24]. Unfortunately, PET was associated with poor sensitivity in the orbit, only identifying lesions in 3 of 11 patients (27%) compared to 8 of 11 on CT or MRI (73%), with the remainder being seen only on physical examination. Other studies have reported higher accuracy in identification of the primary lesion in 15 of 19 eyes (79%) in 16 patients with any type of OAL [25] and 75% of extragastric MALT lymphomas (compared to 39% of gastric MALT) in a study of 33 patients [26]. In 42 patients with MALT lymphomas of any site, sensitivity for the primary site of disease was reported to be 81%; of note, 4 of 6 patients without significant uptake had gastric MALT [27]. Hoffman and colleagues separated MALT lymphomas by their microscopic degree of plasmacytic differentiation and found significant PET avidity in 16 of 19 patients (84%) with plasmacytic differentiation, but only 3 of 16 patients (19%) without [28].

The variability in detection of orbital lesions may be secondary to evolving PET techniques, as MALT lymphomas often arise from a background of inflammation, are generally located in the backdrop of metabolically active extraocular muscles, and have a wide range of tumor histologies seen with different distributions across small clinical series. These include increased baseline metabolic activity and PET signal coming from the extraocular muscles or nearby brain, typically small tumor sizes (particularly after biopsy) and the small size of the orbit (typically encompassing 30 mm³) in combination with a PET resolution of 4–5 mm. Despite these

limitations, the role of PET continues to evolve and improve as a tool for staging and definition of disease. In summary, most series report good sensitivity to systemic disease with the upstaging of some patients beyond conventional imaging (typically 10–20%), but highly variable sensitivity at the primary site.

PET has also shown promise as a tool to evaluate response to therapy in intermediate- and high-grade nodal NHL [29]. If a PET is initially positive in the orbit, this may be used to monitor future disease response as well. In one review of 16 patients with orbital NHL, all 7 patients who underwent post-radiation PET had resolution of pre-treatment increased uptake despite the fact that 3 patients continued to have abnormalities on CT or MRI [25]. PET response to therapy has been documented in other series [26,27], however, these have yet to be correlated to clinical outcome in a large group of MALT lymphoma patients as they have in other body sites. The slow growth of these lesions and the rarity of visual loss caused by tumor progression allows for good clinical follow-up, potentially reducing the impact of PET as a tool for assessing response to therapy.

Somatostatin Receptor Scintography in Staging and Definition of Orbital Disease: A Useful Future Modality

Somatostatin receptor scintography (SRS) using radiolabeled octreotide has found a role in the localization of meningiomas, neuroendocrine tumors, thyroid cancers, Merkel cell carcinoma and other malignancies. SRS has been preliminarily tested for a variety of lymphomas and has significant value in Hodgkin's disease with 98% sensitivity at the sites of documented disease in 56 untreated patients, and was able to detect additional sites of disease missed by conventional imaging in 20 patients (36%). This resulted in change of stage in 12 cases (21%) and change of treatment modality in 7 (13%) [30]. This was confirmed in a larger series of 126 patients revealing a 94% sensitivity, and was notably more effective in diagnosing disease above the diaphragm (98% sensitivity) than below (67%) [31].

When applied to low-grade lymphomas, SRS demonstrated an 84% sensitivity with 20% upstaging and 10% change in treatment plans over conventional imaging alone, in a group of 50 patients [32]. However, SRS imaging was also negative in 38% of lesions identified by conventional imaging. When looking at low-grade lymphoma as a group, the role of SRS, much like PET, is in systemic upstaging with a more limited role in targeting, given high rates of false negatives for particular lesions. Low-grade lymphomas, however, are a heterogeneous group. MALT lymphomas specifically display a pattern of somatostatin receptor expression that may make extragastric MALT uniquely suited to SRS-guided radiotherapy.

To date, five different somatostatin receptor subtypes have been identified and their expression in different tumor types is variable, explaining the differences in the sensitivity and specificity of SRS. Using Northern blot analysis, tissue samples from extragastric MALT were found to strongly express SST_2, while MALT of gastric origin expressed mainly SST_3 and SST_4 [33]. At this point, octreotide SRS relies primarily on SST_2 and SST_5 for binding, however imaging ligands for other receptor subtypes are being sought. The biology fits clinical imaging results perfectly with only 1 of 15 endoscopically confirmed gastric MALT lymphomas demonstrating SRS uptake [33], while a group of 24 patients with extragastric MALT all expressed positive SRS uptake in all known sites of disease [34].

There are data demonstrating the potential superiority of SRS to conventional imaging in assessing response to therapy for patients with extragastric MALT. Thirteen of these extragastric MALT patients also underwent post-therapy SRS scanning with better correlation to clinical outcome than conventional imaging. Seven patients had complete response (CR) and two had persistent disease concordant with conventional imaging. All seven patients with CR on SRS have remained disease-free at 24-month median follow-up. One patient with a liver MALT demonstrated resolution of two of four sites on CT and MRI, even though these sites remained uniformly positive on SRS, a finding which was later confirmed on biopsy as viable lymphoma. In two patients with lacrimal MALT lymphomas, SRS remained positive, while ultrasound and MRI demonstrated resolution of lesions. Both patients relapsed within 9 months. SRS thus appears more reliable than conventional imaging in assessing tumor response post-therapy, at least in the small set of patients that have been studied to date.

In summary, both PET and SRS are useful in the upfront staging of OAL and have been shown to alter stage and treatment recommendations in a number of patients. SRS has an excellent sensitivity for extragastric MALT lymphoma (>90%), both for systemic staging and detection of local disease. This is not the case for gastric MALT as it is rarely detected, and other low-grade lymphomas for which sensitivity is variable. For extragastric MALT, SRS is potentially more accurate than conventional imaging in assessing response to therapy. This may become significant with the addition of more options for therapy, though in an indolent disease this effect will likely be less dramatic. In addition, given the superficial conjunctival location of many orbital MALT lymphomas, these are probably sufficiently followed by examination alone.

Treatment

Observation alone is a consideration for patients with indolent histology OAL, particularly given that visual changes are among the less common symptoms due to the tendency of the disease to mold itself around orbital structures rather than invade. This is exemplified in a Japanese series of 36 patients undergoing observation only [35]. With a median follow-up of 7.1 years, 69% had not required treatment and there were only two deaths associated with lymphoma. High-grade transformation was seen in only one patient. Some, however, would argue that OAL seen in different parts of the world may have variable natural history given potentially different inciting factors.

Recently, there has been major interest in the association of orbital MALT lymphoma and *Chlamydia psittaci* infection. Ferrari et al. found evidence of *C. psittaci* infection in over 80% of DNA samples of patients affected by OAL [36] and propose this as a potential antigenic stimulus. Follow-up clinical trials have shown response rates of 40–60% to a 3-week course of Doxycycline in patients with both localized and systemic disease [37,38]. This association has been controversial and further research is required to confirm and further characterize the role of antibiotics.

Surgical excision and cryotherapy have a limited role in the management of OAL, given the typically diffuse nature of the disease. There are case reports of successful excision or ablation of localized conjunctival lesions, but this should be reserved for

rare circumstances or patients unable to receive other modalities of treatment [39].

Systemic chemotherapy is typically reserved for systemic disease, bilateral disease or aggressive histologies, such as DLBCL. However, there are reports of good response rates for CHOP (cyclophosphamide, adriamycin, vincristine, prednisone), CVP (cyclophosphamide, vincristine, prednisilone) and even single-agent oral chlorambucil in isolated low-grade lesions [40–42]. In one review of 114 patients, radiation therapy was associated with superior local control in comparison to chemotherapy without any difference in overall survival, however this is subject to significant bias in its retrospective nature [43]. A randomized trial demonstrated no benefit in local control, event-free survival or overall survival for the addition of anthracycline-based chemotherapy to 34–40 Gy of radiation therapy in patients with MALT lymphomas [44]. The use of single-agent anti-CD20 antibodies in OAL is an area of emerging research. Efficacy of this agent has been demonstrated in patients with untreated OAL as a single agent, as well as in combination with oral chlorambucil [45–47]. This represents a reasonable emerging option, especially in patients with bilateral disease or risk factors for toxicity with radiation.

Radiation Therapy

Radiation therapy has been the primary mode of definitive therapy for OAL, with excellent rates of disease control and minimal complications of therapy. Techniques of delivery and total dose have varied considerably in the history of OAL.

Radiation Fields

Fields used in the treatment of OAL have included en face AP photon or electron fields, wedged pair arrangements (horizontal or vertical), three-field with wedges, opposed laterals (primarily for bilateral involvement) or, recently, intensity-modulated radiation therapy (IMRT) treatment plans. Typically, lesions confined to the conjunctiva are treated with a single anterior electron field, while retrobulbar lesions require more complex planning with either anterior photons or multiple beams. Fig. 9.1 compares four potential plans: en face electron, en face photon, wedge pair photon and IMRT. In comparing IMRT and wedge pair to en face plans, the advantage is a decreased anterior hot spot with the drawback of greater integral dose. Representative dose volume histograms (DVH) for the conventional plans are shown in Fig. 9.2. Treatment plan and DVH are clearly highly dependent on the anatomy of the patient and tumor, and choice of treatment set-up is typically conducted case by case.

Radiation Dose

A wide range of radiation doses have been reported in the literature. All studies suggest excellent rates of local control within the range of 20–30.6 Gy or higher (see Table 9.2), though there have been some conflicting results as to the ideal dose. Data from aggressive NHL at other sites suggest consideration of doses up to 40 Gy in the absence of a CR with chemotherapy. The difficulty in establishing precise dosage recommendations is likely due to the heterogeneous nature of OAL. This group comprises a wide range of histologies with potentially different causes, from environmental to antigenic to genetic. In addition, due to the relative rarity of OAL, the available data is primarily retrospective

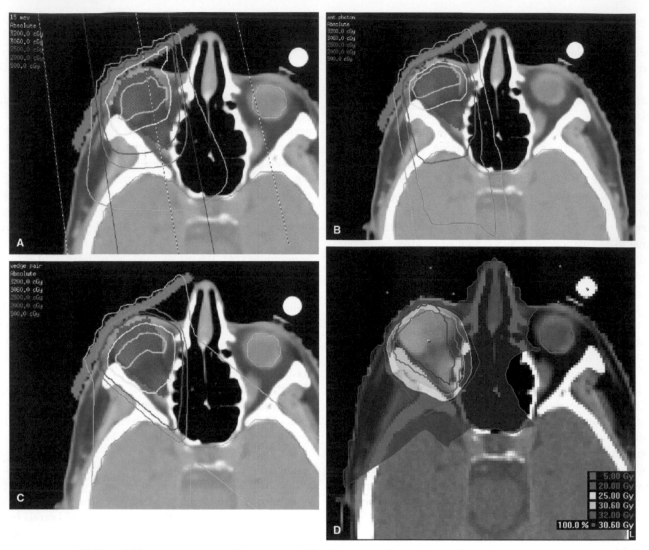

Figure 9.1 A comparison of different field arrangements to treat the same CTV. (A) En face 15 MeV electron beam with 5 mm bolus. (B) En face 6 MV photon beam with 5 mm bolus. (C) Wedge pair 6 MV photon beam with 5 mm bolus. (D) Coplanar IMRT with 6 MV photons.

from large referral centers and, therefore, is subject to significant selection biases.

Most series will suggest that the higher doses approaching 36 Gy are probably more than adequate. A series of 35 treated orbits from Stanford demonstrated no difference in outcome of patients treated with doses of ≤34 Gy compared to those treated with higher doses, also noting measurable vision loss from radiation-related retinal damage in two patients receiving ≥34 Gy [6]. Similarly, Uno et al. demonstrated no increase in local control for doses exceeding 30 Gy [51]. In addition, a series from Taiwan treating 18 patients with 40 Gy was associated with the highest reported cataract rate (35%) and also had a patient requiring corneal transplantation for a recalcitrant ulcer [6]. Given the excellent rates of local control in all series listed in Table 9.2, keeping dose below 34 Gy to limit toxicity seems reasonable.

There is greater debate over whether dose can be lowered below 30 Gy. In a retrospective review of 53 cases of MALT lymphoma receiving a median radiation dose (adjusted by the linear quadratic method to 1.8 Gy per fraction) of 31.8 Gy (range 23.1–45 Gy), Fung et al. described increased local failure with treatment

to <30 Gy; 5-year local control was 81% for the 12 eyes receiving <30 Gy and 100% >30 Gy ($p<0.01$) [12]. Patients with follicular lymphoma histology in the same study achieved 100% local control regardless of treatment dose. Other series, however, have supported lower doses being effective: in a series of 46 patients with 62 orbits treated for OAL, in which 34% of orbits were treated to doses <30 Gy, Zhou et al. reported only one case of local failure [49]. This came in a fairly atypical patient with follicular lymphoma who presented with orbital disease 6 years later at the time of transformation to DLBCL and was therefore at higher risk for local failure than typical OAL patients. Kennerdell reported an excellent 95% rate of local control beyond 5 years in a group of 54 patients treated to 24 Gy, over half of whom had malignant histology lymphomas [52]. A very limited series suggests further reduction in dose may be associated with increased risk of failure; 3 of 11 patients receiving <20 Gy developed failure compared to none receiving >30 Gy [53]. Choosing dose based on histology is further complicated by the uncertainty of histology. The 31 patients with MALT lymphoma reported in a Stanford series were found on a central pathology review of all patients with diagnosis of

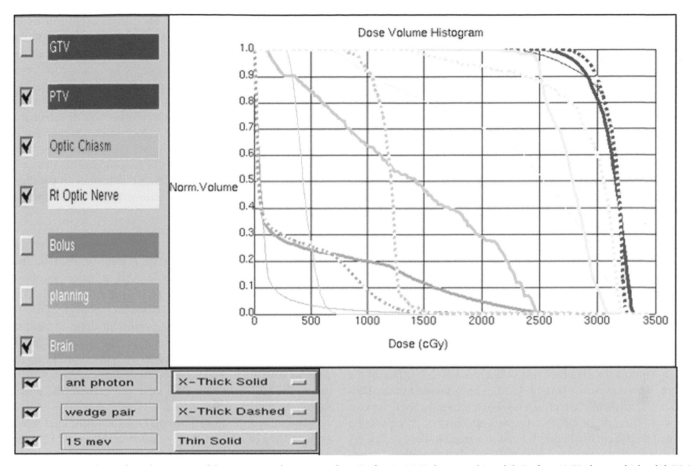

Figure 9.2 Comparative dose-volume histograms of the conventional treatment plans. En face 15 MeV electrons: thin solid. En face 6 MV photon: thick solid. Wedge pair 6 MV photons: dashed.

Table 9.2 Radiation Therapy for Ocular Adnexal Lymphoma

Author	Patients	Eyes	Median dose (Gy)	Dose range	Median FUP	Local control (%)	5-year DSS	5-year OS	Notes
Zhou (Dana-Farber)	46	62	30.6	34% received <30 Gy	46 months	98	98%	88%	63% primary presentation. Overall 48% MALT, 30% follicular
Tsang (Princess Margaret)	30	31	25	All but 1 patient received 25 Gy	61 months	94	n/a	n/a	Data extracted from series of multiple MALT sites
Suh (Yonsei U, Korea)	48	52	30.6	5.4–30.6 Gy, only 2 patients <25.2 Gy	70 months	94	98% (10 years)	87% (10 years)	100% primary orbital MALT
Fung (Mass. General)	98	102	30.6	16.2–46 Gy	82 months	92	75% (45% 10 years)	81% (10 years)	86% primary presentation. Overall 57% MALT, 18% follicular
Uno (Multi-inst, Japan)	50	50	36	20–46 Gy	46 months	94	88%	91%	100% primary orbital MALT
Kennerdell (Allegheny Gen)	54	54	24	24–25.5 Gy	>5 years	95	n/a	n/a	56% malignant lymphomas
Liao (National Taiwan U)	20	20	40	30–40 Gy, 2 patients received 30 Gy	56 months (mean)	100	95%	n/a	68% low grade (includes 5 patients not treated)
Le (Stanford)	31	35	34 (mean)	30–40 Gy	71 months	100	(71% 10 years DFS)	73%	100% MALT (39% MALT, 42% SLL prior to review)

orbital lymphoma, only 12 of whom were initially reported as having MALT histology. At our institution, we typically prescribe 25–30.6 Gy in 1.5–1.8 Gy per fraction, reserving lower doses for patients with a history of dry eye or pre-existing auto-immune or inflammatory disorders.

Lens Blocking

Three techniques for reducing dose to the lens have been commonly used and are associated with lower risk of cataract formation. For anterior electron fields, a simple 10–12 mm diameter central lead shield has been described. Thinner shields of 2–5 mm may be easily mounted to contact lenses. Thicker shields of 2 cm have also been described even in association with contact lenses, but may require more support due to weight on the eye. Thicker shields provide a greater degree of shielding. In early phantom studies, 2.3 mm shields for 6 MeV and 4.3 mm shields for 9 MeV electron beams brought the dose to the lens down to 5–18% of the total tumor dose [48]. Lens shields are contraindicated in tumors that approach the limbus, as this may result in under dosing of portions of the tumor. Hanging eye blocks may be used for photon therapy when there is no tumor extending either directly or in the retrobulbar region behind the block. These typically hang from a support on the block tray and approach the surface of the patient, who is typically immobilized in an Aquaplast mask. Lens blocking is clinically effective and when properly used appears to reduce the rate of cataract formation. Zhou et al. reported a series of 46 patients (62 eyes) treated to a median dose of 30.6 Gy resulting in 9 documented cataracts requiring surgical correction at a median of 37 months after radiation [49]. All of these occurred in patients treated with photons without lens blocking, resulting in a 20% rate of cataract formation in this population. None of the 17 eyes treated with a lens block developed cataracts requiring surgery. Similarly, Fung et al. describe cataracts in 10% of eyes treated by photons without lens shielding at doses ≤32.4 Gy and 36% >32.4 Gy, but only 2 of 45 (4%) treated with electrons and lens shielding [12]. A third technique of lens blocking is only applicable to disease behind the posterior pole of the eye and involves the use of a lateral D-shaped field with split-beam technique, placing the isocenter just posterior to the lens. Placement of an additional lens shield anteriorly in the lateral field does allow for slightly more anterior treatment with anterior displacement of the entire field. Caution must be exercised in selection of patients for lens blocking as cases of tumor recurrence in blocked regions of improperly selected patients have been described [50]. Salvage with radiation or other therapies has been excellent in these cases, but due to refinements in lens replacement surgeries, cataract formation is becoming a less serious side effect.

Focal Radiation Therapy

OAL is frequently a locally multifocal disease. It may occasionally recur in undertreated regions of the eye following improper use of a lens block [50]. Partial orbital irradiation has been examined as a strategy to reduce treatment toxicity; Pfeffer et al. compared 12 patients with limited orbital MALT treated with partial orbital radiation to 11 patients with more extensive lesions treated with whole orbit radiation [54]. Extent of disease was defined by contrast-enhanced thin-sliced CT under Aquaplast immobilization. The acute and long-term toxicities were similar between groups,

and 4 of 12 patients (33%) in the partial orbit arm developed disease recurrence outside of the initial target volume. While there are limited data formally comparing localized versus whole orbit treatments, some authors have described excellent local control in patients with conjunctival lesions treated with a margin, reserving whole orbit radiation for those patients with intra-orbital involvement [49]. Others report on the routine use of lacrimal gland blocking provided this does not block known tumor with good overall local control [52]. However, the results have not been stratified by the focal treatment of conjunctival lesions or use of lacrimal blocks, therefore the precise outcomes in patients with selectively limited fields is not known above the outcome of the group as a whole.

Image-guided Radiation Therapy for Ocular Adnexal Lymphoma

At present, partial orbital radiation remains unproven. The only study comparing partial to whole orbit radiation demonstrated increased rates of failures in the partial orbit group [54]. The comfort level of some authors in treating conjunctival lesions focally with margin may stem from the ability of these to be localized on expert clinical examination. If reliable imaging techniques were better able to guide the delivery of partial orbit radiation in patients with intra-orbital involvement, this may be a viable technique, though margins should take into account the potentially multifocal nature of the disease.

At our institution, we have applied this technique selectively in the setting of a lesion clearly demonstrable on PET in a patient with pre-existing dry-eye, auto-immune or inflammatory disease, in an attempt to reduce the dose delivered to sensitive structures. In such cases, we have fused PET images to CT to define a gross tumor volume (GTV) before adding a margin for planning target volume (PTV). An example is shown in Fig. 9.3. In this case, the anterior orbital GTV is clearly visualized on CT, while the most posterior involvement is ambiguous. The PET helps clarify the posterior extent of the lesion. Definition of the posterior border influences choice of energy and prescription line for anterior photon and electron fields and becomes even more critical if using an IMRT plan. The implications of IMRT plans that do not treat the entire posterior region are not yet known, since this was nearly always treated historically with the use of primarily en face fields. In this case, the majority of the orbit was probably treated with little sparing of structures that may provide lubrication.

While only a subset of OAL patients are PET positive, further verification of the excellent sensitivity of extragastric MALT to SRS may lead to a greater role for the use of IGRT for OAL. SRS may be a better tool for defining the extent of orbital disease. Further study is required to determine whether functional imaging can be used to limit volumes without increasing the risk of orbital recurrence outside the high-dose region. In addition, as low-dose radiotherapy is associated with low baseline morbidity, it remains to be seen whether focal treatment can further reduce morbidity. Another potential approach for those who would choose to treat to higher doses would be to treat the whole orbit as a clinical target volume (CTV) and treat to 20–25 Gy followed by a focal boost to the GTV as defined by examination, conventional imaging and PET/SRS. Again, the difference in toxicity of this strategy compared to treating the whole orbit is unclear given the very modest morbidity of whole orbit treatment to doses around 30 Gy.

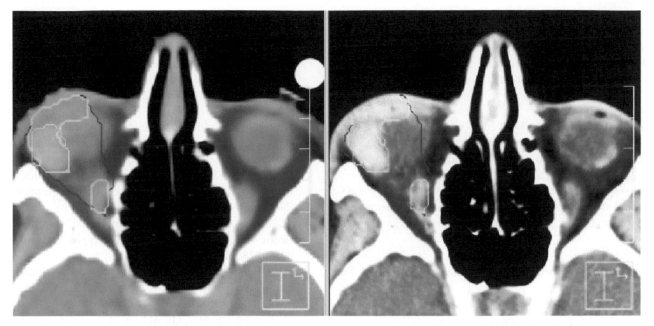

Figure 9.3 Manual fusion of axial CT and PET. Grey contour: volume clearly apparent on CT. Green: volume apparent with PET. Red: combined CTV.

At this point, the role of IGRT in OAL requires further study and should be applied only selectively or in the setting of a protocol.

Re-irradiation

Due to the low doses required for control of OAL, re-irradiation in the case of treatment failure is an option, as well as potential salvage with immunotherapy (i.e., Rituxan) or chemotherapy. Given the rarity of OAL and the excellent local control rates, it is not surprising that no studies have focused specifically on re-irradiation. Successful cases are reported within several larger series or primary treatment. Suh et al. describe three patients with in-orbit failures of MALT lymphomas thought to be due to improper use of lens shielding in otherwise whole-orbit treatments [50]. Failures occurred 34–52 months after initial treatment and were re-treated with whole orbit radiation (26.2–30.6 Gy), bringing the total orbital dose to 53–60.6 Gy. They do not separate re-treatment patients from their group ($n = 48$) for toxicity, but state that only mild periorbital swelling and conjunctivitis was noted in the group with two cataracts, and no keratitis, retinopathy or ongoing requirement for artificial tears. Likewise, Pfeffer et al. demonstrate successful salvage radiation in three patients with MALT lymphoma recurring outside of partial orbit radiation target volumes with whole orbit radiation [54]. Less is known about salvage of patients with recurrences clearly in the high-dose region of the field.

Radiation Tolerance of Normal Orbital Adnexal Structures

Periocular Skin

Typically one sees radiation dermatitis and madarosis within 2 weeks (the time for migration of cells damaged in the proliferating basal layer to the keratinized layer) at a threshold of around 10 Gy (increasing incidence and severity with hypofractionation, patient age, tangential beams and greater previous sun exposure) [55]. Late effects include telangiectasia, atrophy, depigmentation, fibrosis, permanent madarosis and, rarely, induction of second malignancy.

Cornea/Conjunctiva

Mild punctate epithelial erosions may occur at a threshold of around 20–30 Gy and typically resolve in weeks to months. Corneal erythema, photophobia and mild pain may also be seen around this threshold, which may be improved with topical antibiotics and steroids. Mild early xerophthalmia can be seen at a low-dose threshold with 50% ($n = 27/54$) of patients treated to 24–25.5 Gy for OAL developing transient mild xerophthalmia and chemosis, while 33% ($n = 18/54$) reported mild chronic xerophthalmia [52]. These effects are likely mediated by damage to the Meibomian glands (distributed along the distal lid), lacrimal glands and conjunctival surface mucous production. The incidence of late xerophthalmia rises significantly with dose beyond a threshold o f 30 Gy with severe dry eye (defined as corneal opacification, ulceration or vascularization and secondary vision loss) being reported in 0, 30 and 100% of patients receiving doses of <30, 30–45 and >57 Gy respectively, to 1 cm from the anterior surface [56]. Other late corneal effects are rarely seen at doses used for OAL with the typical threshold for symblepharon around 50 Gy for mild scaring and 80–100 Gy for severe scaring. Phthisis bulbi (shrinking of the globe) may be seen beyond 60 Gy [57].

Lens

Cataract formation is a classic deterministic late effect with a threshold of 200 cGy, a TD_{5-5} of 10 Gy and a TD_{50-5} of 18 Gy [58,59]. Rates of cataract formation seen clinically are significantly lower than that predicted by the TD_{50-5} above. The significance of cataract formation continues to decline as cataract surgery improves, though this probably remains slightly more challenging in a radiated eye. Cataract formation was seen in 20% of eyes treated without lens-shielding, but was not seen with shielding in a series of 62 eyes treated at The Dana-Farber Cancer Institute/ Brigham and Women's Hospital [49]. The highest reported rate of cataract formation is 35% in a study from Taiwan utilizing higher doses of radiation (40 Gy) [60].

Neovascular Glaucoma

Neovascular glaucoma should be rare in patients receiving low doses of fractionated radiation therapy in the range given for OAL. Neovascular glaucoma is more commonly seen with uveal melanoma when high anterior chamber doses are given.

Radiation Retinopathy

Radiation retinopathy has a TD_{5-5} of 45 Gy [58] and was not seen in any of the 68 retinas receiving fractionated radiation therapy to doses <45 Gy [61] in one study and thus should be very uncommon with typical doses used for OAL. Occasional cases have been reported, such as one patient receiving 37.8 Gy in 1.8 Gy per fraction developing retinopathy 12 years after therapy with vision deteriorating to 20/200 in the treated eye [6].

REFERENCES

1. YG Adam, HW Farr. Primary orbital tumors. Am J Surg 122(6):726–31, 1971.
2. C Freeman, JW Berg, SJ Cutler. Occurrence and prognosis of extranodal lymphomas. Cancer 29(1):252–60, 1972.
3. CE Margo, ZD Mulla. Malignant tumors of the orbit. Analysis of the Florida Cancer Registry. Ophthalmology 105(1):185–90, 1998.
4. H Demirci, CL Shields, JA Shields, et al. Orbital tumors in the older adult population. Ophthalmology 109(2):243–48, 2002.
5. SE Coupland, L Krause, HJ Delecluse, et al. Lymphoproliferative lesions of the ocular adnexa. Analysis of 112 cases. Ophthalmology 105(8):1430–41, 1998.
6. QT Le, SM Eulau, TI George, et al. Primary radiotherapy for localized orbital MALT lymphoma. Int J Radiat Oncol Biol Phys 52(3):657–63, 2002.
7. TJ Sullivan, K Whitehead, R Williamson, et al. Lymphoproliferative disease of the ocular adnexa: a clinical and pathologic study with statistical analysis of 69 patients. Ophthal Plast Reconstr Surg 21(3):177–88, 2005.
8. LD Sjo, E Ralfkiaer, BR Juhl, et al. Primary lymphoma of the lacrimal sac: an EORTC ophthalmic oncology task force study. Br J Ophthalmol 90(8):1004–9, 2006.
9. SE Coupland, M Hellmich, C Auw-Haedrich, et al. Prognostic value of cell-cycle markers in ocular adnexal lymphoma: an assessment of 230 cases. Graefes Arch Clin Exp Ophthalmol 242(2):130–45, 2004.
10. DM Knowles, FA Jakobiec, L McNally, et al. Lymphoid hyperplasia and malignant lymphoma occurring in the ocular adnexa (orbit, conjunctiva, and eyelids): a prospective multiparametric analysis of 108 cases during 1977 to 1987. Hum Pathol 21(9):959–73, 1990.
11. JP de Boer, RF Hiddink, M Raderer, et al. Dissemination patterns in non-gastric MALT lymphoma. Haematologica 93(2):201–6, 2008.
12. CY Fung, NJ Tarbell, MJ Lucarelli, et al. Ocular adnexal lymphoma: clinical behavior of distinct World Health Organization classification subtypes. Int J Radiat Oncol Biol Phys 57(5):1382–91, 2003.
13. FA Jakobiec, DM Knowles. An overview of ocular adnexal lymphoid tumors. Trans Am Ophthalmol Soc 87:420–42; 1989, discussion 442–24.
14. TE Johnson, DT Tse, GE Byrne Jr, et al. Ocular-adnexal lymphoid tumors: a clinicopathologic and molecular genetic study of 77 patients. Ophthal Plast Reconstr Surg 15(3):171–79, 1999.
15. PA McKelvie, A McNab, IC Francis, et al. Ocular adnexal lymphoproliferative disease: a series of 73 cases. Clin Experiment Ophthalmol 29(6):387–93, 2001.
16. WL White, JA Ferry, NL Harris, et al. Ocular adnexal lymphoma. A clinicopathologic study with identification of lymphomas of mucosa-associated lymphoid tissue type. Ophthalmology 102(12):1994–2006, 1995.
17. C Matteucci, P Galieni, L Leoncini, et al. Typical genomic imbalances in primary MALT lymphoma of the orbit. J Pathol 200(5):656–60, 2003.
18. M Nola, A Lukenda, M Bollmann, et al. Outcome and prognostic factors in ocular adnexal lymphoma. Croat Med J 45(3):328–32, 2004.
19. AL Weber, RL Dallow, RF Oot. Computed tomography of lymphoproliferative disease of the orbit. Report of 50 patients. Acta Radiol Suppl 369:333–36, 1986.
20. JH Yeo, FA Jakobiec, GF Abbott, et al. Combined clinical and computed tomographic diagnosis of orbital lymphoid tumors. Am J Ophthalmol 94(2):235–45, 1982.
21. TJ Sullivan, AA Valenzuela. Imaging features of ocular adnexal lymphoproliferative disease. Eye 20(10):1189–95, 2006.
22. AE Flanders, GA Espinosa, DA Markiewicz, et al. Orbital lymphoma. Role of CT and MRI. Radiol Clin North Am 25(3):601–13, 1987.
23. E Polito, P Galieni, A Leccisotti. Clinical and radiological presentation of 95 orbital lymphoid tumors. Graefes Arch Clin Exp Ophthalmol 234(8):504–9, 1996.
24. AA Valenzuela, C Allen, D Grimes, et al. Positron emission tomography in the detection and staging of ocular adnexal lymphoproliferative disease. Ophthalmology 113(12):2331–37, 2006.
25. I Gayed, MF Eskandari, P McLaughlin, et al. Value of positron emission tomography in staging ocular adnexal lymphomas and evaluating their response to therapy. Ophthalmic Surg Lasers Imaging 38(4):319–25, 2007.
26. C Perry, Y Herishanu, U Metzer, et al. Diagnostic accuracy of PET/CT in patients with extranodal marginal zone MALT lymphoma. Eur J Haematol 79(3):205–9, 2007.
27. KP Beal, HW Yeung, J Yahalom. FDG-PET scanning for detection and staging of extranodal marginal zone lymphomas of the MALT type: a report of 42 cases. Ann Oncol 16(3):473–80, 2005.
28. M Hoffmann, S Wohrer, A Becerer, et al. 18F-Fluorodeoxy-glucose positron emission tomography in lymphoma of mucosa-associated lymphoid tissue: histology makes the difference. Ann Oncol 17(12):1761–65, 2006.
29. J Altamirano, JR Esparza, J de la Garza Salazar, et al. Staging, response to therapy, and restaging of lymphomas with 18F-FDG PET. Arch Med Res 39(1):69–77, 2008.
30. PJ van den Anker-Lugtenburg, EP Krenning, HY Oei, et al. Somatostatin receptor scintigraphy in the initial staging of Hodgkin's disease. Br J Haematol 93(1):96–103, 1996.
31. PJ Lugtenburg, EP Krenning, R Valkema, et al. Somatostatin receptor scintigraphy useful in stage I–II Hodgkin's

disease: more extended disease identified. Br J Haematol 112(4):936–44, 2001.

32. PJ Lugtenburg, B Lowenberg, R Valkema, et al. Somatostatin receptor scintigraphy in the initial staging of low-grade non-Hodgkin's lymphomas. J Nucl Med 42(2):222–29, 2001.

33. M Raderer, J Valencak, F Pfeffel, et al. Somatostatin receptor expression in primary gastric versus nongastric extranodal B-cell lymphoma of mucosa-associated lymphoid tissue type. J Natl Cancer Inst 91(8):716–18, 1999.

34. M Raderer, T Traub, M Formanek, et al. Somatostatin-receptor scintigraphy for staging and follow-up of patients with extraintestinal marginal zone B-cell lymphoma of the mucosa associated lymphoid tissue (MALT)-type. Br J Cancer 85(10):1462–66, 2001.

35. K Tanimoto, A Kaneko, S Suzuki, et al. Long-term follow-up results of no initial therapy for ocular adnexal MALT lymphoma. Ann Oncol 17(1):135–40, 2006.

36. AJ Ferreri, M Guidoboni, M Ponzoni, et al. Evidence for an association between Chlamydia psittaci and ocular adnexal lymphomas. J Natl Cancer Inst 96(8):586–94, 2004.

37. AJ Ferreri, GP Dognini, M Ponzoni, et al. Chlamydia-psittaci-eradicating antibiotic therapy in patients with advanced-stage ocular adnexal MALT lymphoma. Ann Oncol 19(1):194–95, 2008.

38. AJ Ferreri, M Ponzoni, M Guidoboni, et al. Bacteria-eradicating therapy with doxycycline in ocular adnexal MALT lymphoma: a multicenter prospective trial. J Natl Cancer Inst 98(19):1375–82, 2006.

39. CL Shields, JA Shields, C Carvalho, et al. Conjunctival lymphoid tumors: clinical analysis of 117 cases and relationship to systemic lymphoma. Ophthalmology 108(5):979–84, 2001.

40. GJ Ben Simon, N Cheung, P McKelvie, et al. Oral chlorambucil for extranodal, marginal zone, B-cell lymphoma of mucosa-associated lymphoid tissue of the orbit. Ophthalmology 113(7):1209–13, 2006.

41. I Dimitrakopoulos, G Venetis, V Kaloutsi, et al. Effect of chemotherapy on primary mucosa-associated lymphoid tissue lymphoma of the orbit. J Oral Maxillofac Surg 66(1):16–20, 2008.

42. EK Song, SY Kim, TM Kim, et al. Efficacy of chemotherapy as a first-line treatment in ocular adnexal extranodal marginal zone B-cell lymphoma. Ann Oncol 19(2):242–46, 2008.

43. K Tanimoto, A Kaneko, S Suzuki, et al. Primary ocular adnexal MALT lymphoma: a long-term follow-up study of 114 patients. Jpn J Clin Oncol 37(5):337–44, 2007.

44. A Aviles, N Neri, A Calva, et al. Addition of a short course of chemotherapy did not improve outcome in patients with localized marginal B-cell lymphoma of the orbit. Oncology 70(3):173–76, 2006.

45. AJ Ferreri, M Ponzoni, G Martinelli, et al. Rituximab in patients with mucosal-associated lymphoid tissue-type lymphoma of the ocular adnexa. Haematologica 90(11):1578–79, 2005.

46. L Rigacci, L Nassi, M Puccioni, et al. Rituximab and chlorambucil as first-line treatment for low-grade ocular adnexal lymphomas. Ann Hematol 86(8):565–68, 2007.

47. TJ Sullivan, D Grimes, I Bunce. Monoclonal antibody treatment of orbital lymphoma. Ophthal Plast Reconstr Surg 20(2):103–6, 2004.

48. SF Dunbar, RM Linggood, KP Doppke, et al. Conjunctival lymphoma: results and treatment with a single anterior electron field. A lens sparing approach. Int J Radiat Oncol Biol Phys 19(2):249–57, 1990.

49. P Zhou, AK Ng, B Silver, et al. Radiation therapy for orbital lymphoma. Int J Radiat Oncol Biol Phys 63(3):866–71, 2005.

50. CO Suh, SJ Shim, SW Lee, et al. Orbital marginal zone B-cell lymphoma of MALT: radiotherapy results and clinical behavior. Int J Radiat Oncol Biol Phys 65(1):228–33, 2006.

51. T Uno, K Isobe, N Shikama, et al. Radiotherapy for extranodal, marginal zone, B-cell lymphoma of mucosa-associated lymphoid tissue originating in the ocular adnexa: a multi-institutional, retrospective review of 50 patients. Cancer 98(4):865–71, 2003.

52. JS Kennerdell, NE Flores, RJ Hartsock. Low-dose radiotherapy for lymphoid lesions of the orbit and ocular adnexa. Ophthal Plast Reconstr Surg 15(2):129–33, 1999.

53. CK Chao, HS Lin, VR Devineni, et al. Radiation therapy for primary orbital lymphoma. Int J Radiat Oncol Biol Phys 31(4):929–34, 1995.

54. MR Pfeffer, T Rabin, L Tsvang, et al. Orbital lymphoma: is it necessary to treat the entire orbit? Int J Radiat Oncol Biol Phys 60(2):527–30, 2004.

55. CS Hamilton, JW Denham, M O'Brien, et al. Underprediction of human skin erythema at low doses per fraction by the linear quadratic model. Radiother Oncol 40(1):23–30, 1996.

56. JT Parsons, FJ Bova, CR Fitzgerald, et al. Severe dry-eye syndrome following external beam irradiation. Int J Radiat Oncol Biol Phys 30(4):775–80, 1994.

57. SR Durkin, D Roos, B Higgs, et al. Ophthalmic and adnexal complications of radiotherapy. Acta Ophthalmol Scand 85(3):240–50, 2007.

58. B Emami, J Lyman, A Brown, et al. Tolerance of normal tissue to therapeutic irradiation. Int J Radiat Oncol Biol Phys 21(1):109–22, 1991.

59. EJ Hall, AJ Giaccia. Radiobiology for the radiologist. 6th ed. Philadelphia, PA: Lippincott Williams & Wilkins; 2006.

60. SL Liao, SC Kao, PK Hou, et al. Results of radiotherapy for orbital and adnexal lymphoma. Orbit 21(2):117–23, 2002.

61. JT Parsons, FJ Bova, CR Fitzgerald, et al. Radiation retinopathy after external-beam irradiation: analysis of time-dose factors. Int J Radiat Oncol Biol Phys 30(4):765–73, 1994.

10 B-Cell Non-Hodgkin's Lymphoma of the Stomach
Tony Y Eng and Chul S Ha

Introduction

The gastrointestinal (GI) tract is relatively rich in lymphatics and is a major component of the mucosal immune system [1]. There are large numbers of lymphocytes and plasma cells within the mucosa and submucosa of the GI tract, particularly the small bowel and colon. It is the largest immunologic organ in the body and the most common site for extranodal non-Hodgkin's lymphoma (NHL), accounting for up to 20% of all NHL [2]. Although the gastric mucosa is mostly devoid of lymphoid tissue, the stomach is the most frequent site for NHL within the GI tract, representing nearly 50–60% of all GI lymphomas, followed in frequency by small bowel, colon and appendix [3]. Gastric lymphomas comprise mostly low-grade mucosa-associated lymphoid tissue (MALT) lymphomas or diffuse large B-cell lymphomas (DLBCL). Some of these tumors have unique etiologic association with infection by *Helicobacter pylori*. Less frequently, other nodal-type lymphomas (e.g., Burkitt's, mantle cell, follicle center lymphomas) may also present in the GI tract.

Management of primary gastric lymphoma (PGL) remains controversial as there are no consistent clinical trial data available to evaluate the different therapeutic modalities. However, with improving success of systemic chemotherapy and better understanding of the etiology of gastric lymphoma, the management of patients with gastric lymphoma has gradually shifted away from radical surgical management over the past decade, even in many localized cases. At the same time, the role of radiation therapy has changed significantly, not just due to advances in conformal intensity-modulated radiation therapy (IMRT), but also the parallel progress in functional images and image-guided radiation therapy (IGRT) allowing better non-invasive assessment and more accurate treatment delivery. In this chapter, we present the general overview of gastric lymphoma, its pathogenesis and current research endeavors. Although there is a continual lack of consensus in the approach to these tumors, we explore some of the new technologic platforms to assess, plan and execute radiation therapy alone or in coordination with systemic treatment in the management of gastric lymphoma.

Stomach Non-Hodgkin's Lymphoma

PGLs represent approximately 2–9% of gastric tumors in the USA with an apparently increasing incidence worldwide, with higher incidence in Southeast Asia [4–6]. Most studies report a male predominance, mainly of middle-aged Caucasian men, 50–60 years old. The most common histological subtypes are either low-grade MALT-type (30–40%) or high-grade DLBCL (55–60%), of which some may possess a residual low-grade component of MALT (mixed) [7]. Histologically, they appear similar to lymphomas in other sites. MALT lymphoma is a distinct clinical pathologic entity and is considered to be a transformed marginal zone B-cell lymphoma with a smaller number of T-cell lineage under the Revised European–American Lymphoma (REAL) and the World Health Organization (WHO) classification systems as extranodal marginal zone B-cell lymphoma of MALT type [8,9]. Table 10.1 shows the REAL classification of B-cell lymphoma.

Clinical Presentation

The presenting clinical symptoms of gastric lymphoma, like those of gastric adenocarcinoma, are vague, non-specific, gradual and prolonged [10]. The most common complaint is dull epigastric pain resembling peptic ulcer disease or gastritis, often accompanied by weight loss and anorexia that may be the only manifestations present for months or years before the diagnosis is made. This may also be accompanied by dyspepsia, loss of appetite, early satiety, nausea, vomiting and gastric bleeding with guaiac positive stools. A large study of 144 patients suggests persistent vomiting and weight loss may be more frequently present in patients with high-grade lymphoma than in those with low-grade lymphoma [11]. Unlike Hodgkin's lymphoma, overt constitutional symptoms of fever and night sweats are relatively rare, occurring in fewer than 15% of patients. Clinical lymphadenopathy is rare. Although most patients have no physical signs, a palpable abdominal mass may be present in up to one-third of patients at diagnosis. Outlet obstruction, perforation, and fistula formation are uncommon until late in the disease course when the muscular layer is involved [12]. In general, gastric MALT lymphomas are significantly less prone to dissemination than extragastric MALT lymphoma at diagnosis [13].

Risk Factors and Pathogenesis

Common risk factors for gastric lymphoma include *H. pylori* infection, long-term immunosuppression after solid-organ transplantation, celiac disease, inflammatory bowel disease, human immunodeficiency virus (HIV) infection and genetic predisposition [14–17]. Of these, the principal risk factor for the development of gastric MALT lymphoma is infection with *H. pylori*, a microaerophilic, Gram-negative rod. *H. pylori* infection, which may be present in more than 50% of the human population, selectively colonizes gastric mucosa. It is hypothesized that gastric MALT lymphoma develops in the stomach in response to chronic antigenic stimulation from *H. pylori* infection [18], which causes an immunological response, leading to chronic gastritis with formation of lymphoid follicles within the stomach. These lymphoid follicles resemble nodal tissues found throughout the body. These are composed of reactive T cells, activated plasma cells and B cells. The B cells are responsible for initiating a clonal expansion of centrocyte-like cells that form the basic histology of MALT lymphoma. In addition to MALT lymphoma, it also causes gastric ulcer, autoimmune gastritis and other gastric cancer [19].

Underlying immune disorders have been linked to the development of MALT lymphoma, which frequently occurs in women [20]. These patients tend to present at a younger age with mostly extragastric lymphomas and may have a lower response rate to *H. pylori* eradication therapy in the case of gastric lymphoma. However, the

Table 10.1 REAL Classification System: B-cell Neoplasms [8]

B-cell neoplasms

I. Precursor B-cell neoplasm
1. Precursor B-cell lymphoblastic leukemia/lymphoma

II. Mature B-cell neoplasms
1. B-cell chronic lymphocytic leukemia/small lymphocytic lymphoma
2. B-cell prolymphocytic leukemia
3. Lymphoplasmacytic lymphoma
4. Splenic marginal zone lymphoma
5. Hairy cell leukemia
6. Plasma cell myeloma
7. Solitary plasmacytoma of bone
8. Extraosseous plasmacytoma
9. Extranodal marginal zone B-cell lymphoma of mucosa-associated lymphoid tissue (MALT-lymphoma)
10. Nodal marginal zone B-cell lymphoma
11. Follicular lymphoma
12. Mantle cell lymphoma
13. Diffuse large B-cell lymphoma
14. Mediastinal (thymic) large B-cell lymphoma
15. Intravascular large B-cell lymphoma
16. Primary effusion lymphoma
17. Burkitt's lymphoma/leukemia

III. B-cell proliferations of uncertain malignant potential
1. Lymphomatoid granulomatosis
2. Post-transplant lymphoproliferative disorder, polymorphic

overall clinical course does not appear to be significantly different from MALT lymphoma in patients without underlying immune disorders. To the contrary, PGL is uncommon in HIV-infected patients [21–23]. In most cases of gastric lymphoma in HIV-infected patients, gastric involvement is secondary to advanced extragastric, often multifocal lymphomas. Only a few cases of true PGLs that are limited to the stomach and perigastric nodes without spleen, liver, bone marrow or peripheral blood involvement are reported in the literature [24,25]. Their prognosis is generally poor [26,27].

In patients whose disease is not related to *H. pylori* or chronic inflammation, several recurrent cytogenetic alterations have been reported [28]. Some of these include the trisomies 3 and 18, and the translocations t(11;18)(q21;q21), t(1;14)(p22;q32), t(14;18) (q32;q21), t(3;14)(q27;q32) and t(3;14)(p14.1;q32), of which the most common in MALT lymphomas is a balanced translocation between chromosomes 11 and 18, resulting in the generation of a fusion protein (apoptosis inhibitor-API2-MALT1 fusion product), aberrant nuclear Bcl-10 expression, and activation of the NF-kB pathway [29]. Patients with t(11;18)(q21;q21) translocation may be more likely to develop multifocal disease, whereas patients with both t(11;18)(q21;q21) and Bcl-10 nuclear expression tend to present with more advanced disease and are typically unresponsive to *H. pylori* eradication therapy, requiring more systemic cytotoxic therapy [13]. Approximately 50% of the *H. pylori* independent-MALT lymphomas show the translocation t(11;18)(q21;q21) marker. Other genomic alterations, like trisomy 3 and 18, translocation involving the FOXP1 gene or over-expression of CARMA1 and CARD9 may be associated with the pathogenesis and progression of gastric B-cell lymphoma [30,32].

Pattern of Spread
Although most gastric MALT lymphomas remain clinically localized in 60–70% of patients at presentation (stage I or II disease), they

have a potential to transform to and disseminate like high-grade DLBCL [33,34]. Nodal metastases can occur in 63% of the patients with gastric DLBCL, including the perigastric nodes along the lesser and greater curvature, nodes located along the left gastric, common hepatic, splenic and celiac arteries. The incidence of adjacent organ infiltration by PGL ranges between 7 and 29% in different reports, with the most common sites being the pancreas, omentum and spleen [35–37]. The colon is occasionally involved, and the literature describes a few case reports of gastrocolic fistulae secondary to PGL. Most cases develop in patients with advanced disease and a history of gastric damage. In patients with advanced PGL, disease may potentially spread to extra-intestinal sites, including the liver, kidneys, ovary, and extra-abdominal sites, like the central nervous system, bone and lungs [34,38].

Diagnosis and Workup
The criteria for PGL include tumor arising predominantly in the stomach, with adenopathy, if present, corresponding to the expected lymphatic drainage of the stomach, limited to perigastric nodes without spleen, liver, bone marrow or peripheral blood involvement [39]. Associated involvement of peripheral and mediastinal nodes, bone marrow, liver or spleen may suggest secondary gastric involvement and often precludes the diagnosis of PGL. The pathologic diagnosis of gastric lymphoma is most frequently established by means of endoscopy with multiple biopsies. Endoscopically, compared with high-grade lymphomas that are more frequently ulcerative, low-grade lymphomas are more likely to present as "normal" appearing mucosa or petechial hemorrhage in the fundus, confined to the antrum (stage I) and be associated with *H. pylori* infection [11]. The tumor can have a multifocal distribution, and therefore aggressive tissue sampling is crucial for diagnosis. All pathology slides should be reviewed by an experienced hematopathologist. Histology may show a predominance of centrocyte- or centroblast-like cells, characterized by lymphoid hyperplasia and infiltrations of lymphocytes into glandular epithelium or lymphoepithelial lesions with CD20 expression. The presence of B-cell proliferation, lymphoepithelial lesions, cytologic atypia and Dutcher bodies help make the diagnosis of low-grade MALT lymphoma, while the presence of germinal centers, acute inflammation and reactive epithelial atypia do not exclude a diagnosis of low-grade gastric lymphoma [40]. *H. pylori* infection can be detected with modified Giemsa staining. Identification of t(11;18) by reverse transcription-polymerase chain reaction (RT-PCR) procedure may aid in the diagnosis of gastric MALT lymphoma and also helps predict resistance to *H. pylori* eradication therapy [41]. In addition to pathologic confirmation, PCR procedure may become useful in monitoring molecular evidence of clonal residual after therapy and determining the necessity and length of further treatment [42].

Workup studies include a comprehensive blood count, a lactate dehydrogenase (LDH) level, a comprehensive chemistry panel and a urine analysis. Often, a bone marrow biopsy should also be done. Barium swallow studies can frequently reveal the lesion in a high percentage of cases. Computed tomography (CT) of the chest, abdomen and pelvis is recommended to rule out metastasis. Use of proper contrast materials and optimal timing of its administration are crucial in obtaining good CT images to provide information about the gastric wall and the extent of disease penetration. Various CT patterns may be seen. Some of the

CT features of PGL are clefts and tracks, diffuse or limited wall thickening, lymphadenopathy, rugal prominence and solitary or multiple intraluminal masses [43,44]. Of these, the most common feature seen on CT is gastric wall thickening. Fig. 10.1 illustrates the CT appearance of a primary gastric MALT lymphoma. Fig. 10.2 demonstrates the endoscopic appearance of the same lesion in the fundus. Although the endoscopic appearance of this tumor is varied and can be diffuse, infiltrative, exophytic or ulcerative, endoscopic ultrasonography (EUS) is essential to document the extent of disease and may be more accurate than CT scan in detection of depth of invasion and spread to perigastric lymph nodes [45]. It has been shown to be quite accurate in the evaluation of gastric wall infiltration by lymphoma [46].

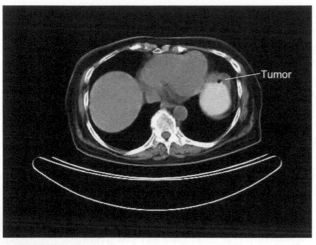

Figure 10.1 Axial CT image showing the abnormal thickening of the gastric wall.

Functional Imaging

Unlike conventional X-rays, CT, magnetic resonance imaging (MRI) and ultrasound, functional or molecular imaging, particularly positron emission tomography (PET), PET-CT and MR spectroscopy (MRS) provide quantitative and metabolic information in addition to anatomical detection of the presence or absence

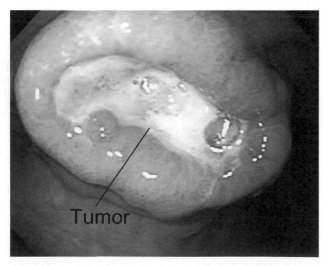

Figure 10.2 Endoscopic appearance of an ulcerative, exophytic gastric MALT lymphoma.

of malignant processes. The entire body, for instance, can be imaged non-invasively, and metabolic activity-directed biopsy can be performed. However, the sensitivity, specificity and accuracy have not been established in PGL. The subjectivity in interpretation and effects of heterogeneity are still problematic. There are very limited data on MRS as it is technically challenging. Nevertheless, non-invasive functional imaging with PET scan can be very useful in staging and guiding therapy in malignant lymphoma. In a small study of 15 patients with gastric lymphoma, the ^{18}F-fluorodeoxyglucose (^{18}F-FDG)-PET scan was positive in all cases of gastric lymphoma with known active disease and negative in all cases with complete clinical remission after treatment [47]. The intensity of ^{18}F-FDG uptake was also higher in aggressive gastric NHL than in MALT lymphoma. Similarly, Phongkitkarun and associates studied 33 patients with biopsy-proven GI NHL, who had undergone ^{18}F-FDG-PET scan before and after treatment [48]. High-grade tumors demonstrated higher intensity of ^{18}F-FDG uptake than that seen in low-grade lesions. As expected, the stomach was identified as the most common primary site of involvement (20 patients). The mean standardized uptake value (SUV) was 3.02 in low-grade gastric MALT lymphoma. The average SUV decreased from 11.58 to 2.21 after treatment in patients with high-grade disease and negative biopsies. ^{18}F-FDG-PET scan appears to help diagnosis, staging or re-staging of disease prior to treatment or to monitor disease response and recurrence or transformation during follow up. Whole body ^{18}F-FDG-PET findings can confirm the extranodal primary origin in the stomach by showing no evidence of distant nodal or non-nodal metastasis [49].

Although specific data on gastric lymphoma are lacking, PET integrated with CT (PET/CT) offers better accuracy and anatomical localization over PET or CT alone in patients with MALT lymphoma and can directly guide biopsies or surgical interventions. Fig. 10.3 illustrates an abnormal uptake corresponding to CT findings. Patient-based evaluation has shown a sensitivity of 78% for CT alone, 86% for ^{18}F-FDG-PET alone and 93% for combined ^{18}F-FDG-PET/CT imaging [50]. In a study of 62 patients with PGL, ^{18}F-FDG-PET/CT was positive in 38/38 (100%) of patients with high-grade gastric lymphoma, whereas it was positive in only 17/24 (71%) patients with low-grade gastric MALT lymphoma [51]. Overall, 89% of patients with PGL were detected by ^{18}F-FDG-PET/CT and tumor uptake of ^{18}F-FDG could be differentiated from physiologic stomach uptake by intensity. In 33 patients with biopsy-proven MALT lymphoma (18 stomach primary), Perry et al. reported better sensitivity in patients with non-gastric advanced disease [52]. The PET/CT sensitivity was only 39% in gastric MALT lymphomas, compared with 75% in non-gastric MALT lymphomas. PET/CT detected active disease only in 42% of the patients with early-stage disease (I–II), but in 100% patients with advanced disease (stage III–IV). Overall, the authors still found PET/CT useful in initial staging and follow-up after therapy in patients with MALT lymphoma.

The improved accuracy of pathologic diagnosis by endoscopic biopsies, coupled with advanced imaging with endoscopic ultrasound, and PET and PET/CT have eliminated the necessity for surgical laparotomy for the diagnosis and staging of gastric lymphoma.

Pathology

Some of the common histologies of PGL include mantle cell lymphoma (malignant lymphomatous polyposis), enteropathy-

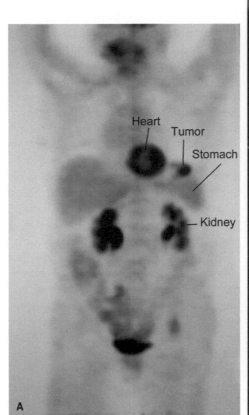
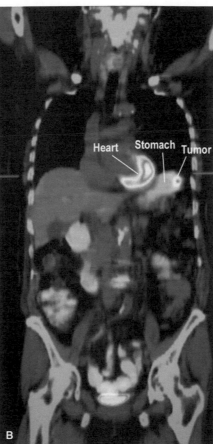

Figure 10.3 (A) PET. (B) PET-CT, AP view showing the corresponding abnormal FDG uptake in the gastric wall.

associated T-cell lymphoma, DLBCL and MALT lymphoma, the latter of which is perhaps the best understood. Gastric lymphoma may appear as small mucosal ulcerations to large fungating polypoidal masses or diffuse multifocal infiltration. PGL most frequently occurs in the distal portion of the stomach, with occasional direct involvement of the duodenum or the distal esophagus. It originates from the lymphoid tissue, predominantly of the B cells, in the lamina propria. Some investigators propose that most lesions are preceded by chronic inflammation and immunostimulation secondary to the antigenic effect of *H. pylori* [53–55]. MALT lymphoma is a distinct disease with specific clinical and pathologic features that may affect diverse organs. While it remains commonly localized within the stomach at presentation, it invades outward through the muscularis and serosa with approximately two-thirds of patients presenting with stage I and II disease and/or regional nodal metastases. Small foci of lymphoid follicles surrounded by neoplastic marginal zone B cells may be found throughout the gastric mucosa at various distances from the main confluent tumor mass [56]. This phenomenon may account for the local relapse within the gastric stump after complete resection with negative microscopic margins. While gastric MALT lymphomas are commonly regarded as low-grade lesions, some pathologists have used the term "high-grade MALT lymphoma" to denote transformation of a low-grade MALT lymphoma. The WHO classification, however, recommends that primary large-cell lymphomas of MALT sites should be diagnosed as diffuse large B-cell lymphoma, not as high-grade MALT lymphoma [57]. Clinically, MALT lymphoma

is an indolent extranodal lymphoma that tends to remain localized with a high potential for cure with local therapy. Morphologically, MALT lymphoma recapitulates the structure of the Peyer's patch [58]. The key difference is based on the presence or absence of histologic features suggestive of MALT lymphoma, including the typical lymphoepithelial lesions with lymphoid follicles and infiltration of characteristic centrocyte-like plasma cells, which have small, dense, granular nuclei with clear cytoplasm and irregular borders. The presence of these histologic features in patients with primary large-cell gastric lymphoma may also be associated with a better response to systemic chemotherapy and a better prognosis [59]. Fig. 10.4 illustrates some of the histologic features of gastric MALT lymphoma. The pivotal feature is the presence of lymphoepithelial lesions arising from centrocyte-like neoplastic B cells infiltrating residual glands.

Staging and Prognostic Factors

Staging

Several staging systems have been employed to stage PGL. Of these, the most commonly applied is a modification of the Ann Arbor staging system for lymphoma, as presented in Table 10.2 [60]. Technically, multifocal or diffuse disease as in disseminated involvement of one or more extralymphatic organs should be assigned stage IV. Clinically, however, this must be distinguished from other advanced disease with multiorgan involvement or bone marrow involvement. Therefore, direct spread of a lymphoma into adjacent tissues or organs does not influence stage and multifocal

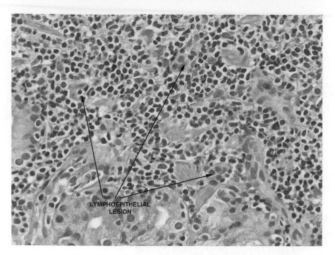

Figure 10.4 Histologic features on H&E 400× of MALT gastric lymphoma characterized by a proliferation of small lymphoid cells with irregularly shaped nuclei and abundant cytoplasm, i.e., centrocyte-like cells, and the presence of lymphoepithelial lesions.

involvement of a single extralymphatic organ is still classified as stage IE, whereas involvement of two or more segments of the GI tract, isolated and not in continuity, is classified as stage IV.

Prognostic Factors
Unlike MALT lymphomas in the small or large intestine, in which no specific treatable etiologic agents have been identified, gastric MALT lymphomas have a better prognosis than their counterparts arising from non-gastric locations [61]. Gastric MALT lymphomas tend to be localized for a long period of time, often stage I and II at presentation and low grade. Even for patients with high-grade gastric DLBCL, the presence of MALT histologic features may confer a better response to systemic chemotherapy and a better prognosis [59]. The most consistent and independent prognostic factors for PGL are stage and grade of the disease [4,35,60]. The 5-year survival for stage I and II patients with PGL was 87 and 61%, respectively [35]. The 5-year survival for patients with low-grade and high-grade PGL was 91 and 56%, respectively. Other adverse factors include depth of invasion through serosa, older age (>60), T-cell histology, a higher index of cell proliferation (Ki-67 or MIB1), elevated LDH, poor performance status, high International Prognostic Index (IPI) and aneuploid lymphoma [62–66]. One study suggests that Epstein-Barr virus (EBV) infection may be a predictive factor for chemotherapy and radiotherapy resistance in diffuse large B-cell gastric lymphoma [67].

Table 10.2 The Musshoff's Staging for Gastric Lymphomas [60]

Stage	Sites of involvement
IE	Tumor confined to the GI tract
IIE1	Tumor with regional nodal involvement (i.e., celiac)
IIE2	Tumor with extra-regional subdiaphragmatic nodal involvement (i.e., para-aortic, iliac, etc.)
IIIE	Tumor with nodal involvement on both sides of the diaphragm
IV	Distant involvement (i.e., bone marrow, lungs, liver, spleen, etc.)

(Modified Ann Arbor Staging System)

Treatment
Antibiotics
Treatment of PGL has been based largely on the stage of disease. Both surgery and non-surgery regimens have been used. Most cases of low-grade primary lymphoma that are confined to the mucosa or submucosa of the gastric wall are believed to be associated with *H. pylori* stimulation and have an indolent course. These patients tend to have stage I or II disease and antibiotics alone can induce complete remissions in these patients. After successful eradication of the infection, these tumors may regress completely and permanently, with complete remission rates ranging from 50 to 100% [68–70]. Therefore, antibiotic regiments should be the first-line therapy for patients with MALT lymphoma associated with *H. pylori* infection or any superficial low-grade MALT lymphoma suspicious of *H. pylori* association. Triple therapy, consisting of a proton pump inhibitor, clarithromycin and amoxicillin, is very effective for the eradication of *H. pylori* infection [68]. It is recommended for the treatment of the superficial type of low-grade gastric MALT lymphoma. Another common antibiotic regiment includes amoxicillin, metronidazole and bismuth, or omeprazole. With proper antibiotic therapy, the *H. pylori* eradication and lymphoma regression rates are well over 80% [71,72]. Unfortunately, the *H. pylori* eradication rates have been decreasing slowly, in part due to increasing antibiotic resistance [73]. Non-progressive, asymptomatic residual local disease after successful eradication of *H. pylori* infection can be managed with careful surveillance. The disease course of these patients tends to remain indolent [74]. Primary gastric MALT lymphomas that are not responsive to antibiotic therapy should be treated with radiation therapy with or without chemotherapy [75–77].

Surgery
Historically, surgery was believed to optimize local disease control and reduce risk of perforation or bleeding. Surgery has played a central role in diagnosis, staging and treatment of this disease with superior outcome in those presented with early stage of disease. Nakamura et al. [78] reported 10-year survival rates of 87 and 60% for stage I and II disease, respectively, in 161 patients with operable PGL following surgical resection. Caronna and associates also reported low mortality and morbidity in a series of 37 patients undergoing radical gastrectomy and D2 lymphadenectomy for stage I and II primary gastric B-cell lymphoma [79]. They compared postoperative histopathological findings to preoperative staging data and found a high incidence of mixed grading of tumors and a relatively high incidence of lymph node metastases in low-grade lymphoma. The investigators advocated systematic primary surgery in PGL as it provides more accurate staging and seems to be curative in stage IE disease. The concern was that relying on preoperative biopsies and imaging techniques could lead to inaccurate staging and inappropriate treatment. If surgery is utilized, most prefer functional subtotal gastrectomy to total gastrectomy or more radical resections when the gross negative margins can be obtained. Positive microscopic margins can be managed with adjuvant therapy. In a prospective, randomized, multicenter study, marginal status did not influence survival, relapse or disease-free survival when all patients received adjuvant therapy [80].

Over the past decade, cumulative data have gradually emerged supporting a more conservative non-surgical approach with chemotherapy with or without radiotherapy as the treatment of choice for PGL, reserving surgery for selected patients, who experience bleeding, perforation or obstruction that does not resolve with non-surgical therapy [81,82]. Primary surgical therapy in these patients may lead to significant risk of complications and delay in initiating systemic therapy. In a large multicenter trial involving 185 patients with stage I or II gastric lymphoma, surgical treatment consisting of gastrectomy with adjuvant whole abdominal radiation therapy with or without chemotherapy was not better than non-surgical treatment with chemotherapy and radiation therapy [64]. The overall 5-year survival rates were 82.5 and 84%, respectively. Hemorrhage occurred in one patient who was treated with chemotherapy only. Another large clinical trial also showed a similar low incidence of hemorrhage and no survival advantage with surgery over non-surgery treatment [81]. In summary, surgery has a very limited role in the management of PGL beyond biopsy.

Chemotherapy

PGLs have been treated successfully with organ-conservative chemotherapy with or without radiation therapy [81–87]. Chemotherapy, in particular the CHOP regimen (cyclophosphamide, doxorubicin, vincristine, prednisone), appears effective in the treatment of PGL, especially for patients with high-grade disease. Conservative treatment with primary doxorubicin-based chemotherapy followed by involved-field radiation therapy should be used as the first-line treatment for patients with early-stage PGL. The response rates range between 70 and 100% and the stomach preservation rates are well over 90% with similar survival as surgery [88–91].

The CHOP regimen is the most effective and frequently used regimen (see Table 10.3). Using a prospectively accrued database, the Royal Marsden Hospital reported their experience with 37 patients with intermediate- or high-grade PGL who received chemotherapy alone or after surgery, from 1985 to 1996. The 5-year overall survival for localized and advanced PGL was 94 and 50%, respectively. There were no differences between the 13 patients who received surgery and the 24 patients who received chemotherapy alone. Furthermore, no perforations or serious bleeding occurred [92]. In a study of 25 patients with stage IE and IIE high-grade PGL who were treated with CHOP alone, chemotherapy achieved a complete remission rate of 96% [85]. Treatment with CHOP was associated with a 2-year overall survival rate of 88%.

In a large treatment comparison study involving 589 patients with early-stage DLBCL PGL (IE and II$_1$) randomized to surgery, surgery plus radiotherapy, surgery plus CHOP chemotherapy, or CHOP chemotherapy alone, Aviles et al. [81] reported 10-year event-free survival rates of 28% for surgery, 23% for surgery plus radiotherapy, 82% for surgery plus chemotherapy and 92% for chemotherapy alone. The corresponding overall 10-year survival rates were 54, 53, 91 and 96%, respectively. Furthermore, surgical treatment was associated with more severe toxicity, with 28 patients dying from surgical complications and 52 patients with "dumping syndrome", whereas no patient died from chemotherapy or radiation therapy complications. In multivariate analysis, the authors found only the type of treatment to be a significant factor for survival outcomes. Thus, it appears that chemotherapy should be considered the treatment of choice in patients with stage IE and IIE primary gastric diffuse large-cell lymphoma.

For patients with locally advanced (stage III) or disseminated (stage IV) gastric lymphoma, primary systemic chemotherapy, with or without radiation or surgery, appears to be optimal [93]. Long-term remission and cure can be achieved and may salvage a proportion of patients with inoperable tumors, especially for cases of high-grade tumors that typically are more sensitive to chemotherapy.

In some recent studies, rituximab (R), the anti-CD20 monoclonal antibody, has either been added to standard chemotherapy, CHOP, or used alone in treating PGL with promising results [94–96]. In 15 patients with early-stage gastric DLBCL, primary treatment with R-CHOP resulted in a complete remission rate of 87% and a partial remission rate of 13% [94]. Similarly, a study of 26 patients with relapsed/refractory gastric MALT lymphoma showed a 77% objective response rate (46% complete pathological response and 31% partial response) with weekly rituximab treatment [95]. The presence of t(11;18)(q21;q21) translocation did not affect the response or subsequent relapse. Rituximab, either as monotherapy or combined therapy (R-CHOP), appears to be effective for patients with gastric MALT lymphoma. R-CHOP has the potential to become the standard chemotherapy for gastric B-cell lymphoma.

Radiation Therapy

Adjuvant and definitive radiation therapy for PGL has been used successfully in some series, resulting in long-term remissions. The Memorial Sloan-Kettering Cancer Center reported an update of 51 patients with MALT lymphoma of the stomach treated with radiation alone [97,98]. The patients had stage I–II$_2$ low-grade PGL without evidence of *H. pylori* infection or with persistent lymphoma after antibiotic therapy for associated *H. pylori* infection. The median total radiation dose was 30 Gy delivered in 1.5-Gy daily fractions to the stomach and adjacent lymph nodes. The 5-year freedom from treatment failure, overall survival and cause-specific survival were 89, 83, and 100%, respectively. Lin et al. [99] reported a complete response rate of 94% on post-radiation endoscopic biopsies in 18 patients with low-grade gastric lymphoma characterized as residual disease (44%), recurrent or progressive (17%) and improving but persistent (28%) after various prior treatments, including *H. pylori* eradication, chemotherapy or surgery. The median radiation dose was 30 Gy. Although recurrence rate was 18%, radiation therapy is an effective, well-tolerated treatment for patients with low-grade PGL, including those who have had prior therapy. The authors and other investigators advocate the use of radiotherapy alone for gastric MALT lymphoma not associated with *H. pylori* infection or tumors not responsive to eradication of the *H. pylori* infection. Similar results have been documented by other investigators in treating MALT lymphoma of the stomach with radiation alone [100,101].

Best Treatment Approach and Treatment Results

Although not widely accepted in the USA, gastrectomy with adjuvant chemotherapy (CHOP) followed by radiotherapy is a common practice for patients with large B-cell stomach lymphoma in Japan, where the incidence of PGL is higher [90,102]. Surgical findings from gastric resection can provide more sufficient material for accurate histopathological diagnosis and clinico-pathological staging, adequacy of extirpation of the tumor, and

Table 10.3 Summary of Selected Treatment Results for Gastric Lymphoma

Authors/year	No. of patients	Stage/histology	Treatment (No. of patients)	Results	Comments
Aviles et al. (2004)[81] randomized	589	IE IIE$_1$ DLBC	Surg (148) Surg+RT 40 Gy (138) Surg+CHOP (153) CHOP (150)	28%, 54% (DFS, OS 10 yr) 23%, 53% 82%, 91% 92%, 92% $P = <0.001$	Largest randomized study. CT was same or better than surgery. Non-surgical treatment is recommended. RT=20 Gy WAR+20 Gy IFRT
Aviles et al. (2006)[82] randomized	102	IE IIE$_1$ HG MALT	Surg+CEOP-Bleo (52) CEOP-Bleo (49)	94%, 70%, 78% (CR, DFS, OS 5 yr) 96%, 67%, 76%	Organ-preserving treatment is effective
Binn et al. (2003)[86]	106	IE IIE DLBC	Surg+CHOP (48) CHOP±RT (58)	91%, 86% (OS, EFS 5 yr) 91%, 92%	International Prognostic Index (IPI) was an independent factor. Similar 5-year survival rates (>90%)
Cogliatti et al. (1991)[35]	145	IE IIE LG and HG	Surg (80) Surg+CT (33) Surg+RT (22) Surg+CT+RT (10)	87% (OS 5 yr, stage I) 61% (stage II) 91% (LG) 56% (HG)	Retrospective, grade and stage were prognostic
Fischbach et al. (2000)[117]	236	IE IIE LG and HG	LG: ABX±Surg±WAR 30+10 Gy boost (97) HG: Surg+CHOP ×6±IFRT 40 Gy (139)	89–96% (OS 2 yr for LG) 83–88% (HG, no gross residual disease) 53% (HG, gross residual disease)	Grade and residual disease after surgery were prognostic factors
Ishikura et al. (2005)[90] Phase II	52	IE IIE HG	CHOP+IFRT 40.5 Gy (52)	92%, 88%, 94% (CR, PFS, OS 2 yr)	Organ-preserving treatment is effective
Koch et al. (2001)[64] GMSG prospective multicenter study	185	IE IIE$_1$ IIE$_2$ LG and HG	Surg+EFRT (WAR) 30±10 Gy boost (79) *COP+EFRT 30+10 Gy boost (106) *For HG: CHOP ×4+EFRT (Stage I) or CHOP ×6+IFRT 40 Gy (Stage II)	84%, 79% (OS, EFS 5 yr) 82%, 79%	Survival was better after complete resection than incomplete resection; overall data favor non-surgical approaches
Koch et al. (2005)[107] GMSG non-randomized study	393	IE IIE HG and LG	Surg±EFRT 30±10 Gy boost (61) *COP+EFRT 30+10 Gy boost (332) *For HG: CHOP ×6+IFRT 30–40 Gy	86%, 83% (OS, EFS at 42 months) 91%, 86%	This study confirmed initial findings that non-surgical approach was equivalent to surgery with same survival rates
Park et al. (2006)[91] PII study	50	IE IIE HG DLBC	CHOP ×4+IFRT 40 Gy (50)	92%, 92%, 92% (CR, PFS, OS 2 yr)	Organ-preserving treatment is effective
Thieblemont et al. (2003)[115]	48	IE IIE LG MALT	Surg (21) Surg+CT±RT (8) Single or CHOP CT (19)	95%, 86% (CR, PFS 5 yr) 100%, 95% 84%, 81%	Similar outcome in patients treated with surgery or CT
Valicenti et al. (1993)[116]	77	IE IIE Mostly DLBC	RT 41–45 Gy (7) CHOP or CVP (11) Surg (12) Surg RT±CHOP (47)	52% (DFS 5 yr) 65% (multimodality) 24% (single modality)	74% of relapses were local. Tumor size ≤5 cm was prognostic; surg+RT had best DFS
Yahalom et al. (2002)[97]	51	IE IIE (*H. pylori* refractory)	IFRT 30 Gy (51)	96% (CR) 89% (FFF 4 yr) 100% (CSS 4 yr)	Excellent RT alone data for gastric MALT lymphomas

Yr: year; Surg: surgery; CT: chemotherapy; RT: radiation therapy; IFRT: involved-field radiation therapy; WAR: whole abdominal radiation; ABX: antibiotics; LG: low grade; HG: high grade; DFS: disease-free survival; CR: complete response; PFS: progression-free survival; EFS: event free survival; CSS: cause-specific survival; FFF: freedom from failure; OS: overall survival; CEOP-Bleo: cyclophosphamide, epirubicin, vincristine, prednisone, bleomycin; CHOP: cyclophosphamide, vincristine, doxorubicin, prednisone; CVP: cyclophosphamide, vincristine, prednisone.

thus better determination of further adjuvant therapy if necessary. However, significant surgical complications may range between 8 and 18% [103–105].

Following their initial German multicenter study of 185 cases of PGL [64,106], Koch et al. [107] reported the results of a subsequent larger, non-randomized study of 393 patients with PGL, confirming their initial results that non-surgical approach was equivalent to surgery. The survival rate at 42 months for patients treated with surgery was 86% compared with 91% for patients treated without surgery. Aviles et al. [81] reported the largest randomized study of 589 patients with stage IE and IIE₁ primary gastric diffuse large-cell lymphoma to evaluate the different treatment modalities. The treatment arms were surgery (148 patients), surgery and 40 Gy of radiation (138 patients), surgery and CHOP chemotherapy (153 patients) and CHOP chemotherapy alone (150 patients). Complete response rates were similar in all four arms. The 10-year actuarial event-free survival rates were 28, 23, 82 and 92%, respectively ($p<0.001$). The corresponding 10-year overall survival rates were 54, 53, 91 and 96% ($p<0.001$). Surgery was noted to be associated with some cases of lethal complications. These studies have established a non-surgical approach, chemotherapy±radiation, as the treatment of choice in patients with PGL, especially high-grade DLBC histology.

Patients with stage I and II gastric MALT lymphoma and *H. pylori* infection should be treated with antibiotics. Those who are not infected with *H. pylori* or don't respond to antibiotics are best treated with radiation therapy alone. Systemic chemotherapy should be the treatment of choice for patients with stage III and IV gastric MALT lymphoma and DLBCL with or without involved-field radiation therapy. Table 10.3 summarizes some of the selected treatment results from studies with a large number of patients. The overall survival rates range 70–100% for patients with stage I and II disease.

Radiation Treatment Planning

Gross Tumor Volume, Clinical Target Volume, Internal Target Volume and Planning Target Volume

There is no consensus on the radiation treatment volume for PGL. Some approaches have used the "traditional fields" originally designed for gastric carcinoma delivering 30–35 Gy to the stomach, whereas others have even employed low-dose, 20–30 Gy, to the whole abdomen effectively followed by a 10–20 Gy boost [64,81]. Involved fields advocated by various investigators are widely different. But commonly, involved field is the entire stomach, including the adjacent lymph nodes.

The clinical target volume (CTV) is defined as the gross tumor volume (GTV) plus any clinically and radiographically suspicious adjacent or regional lymph nodes at risk, including perigastric, celiac, local para-aortic (level L2–3), splenic, hepatoduodenal or hepatic portal, and pancreaticoduodenal nodes. As PGL is often diffuse and multifocal, the CTV should include the entire stomach containing the GTV or residual tumor if after surgery or chemotherapy or tumor bed if no gross disease after primary therapy. The planning target volume (PTV) is defined as the CTV plus an approximately 2–3 cm margin in all directions as appropriate and must be tailored individually. The radiation field should be based

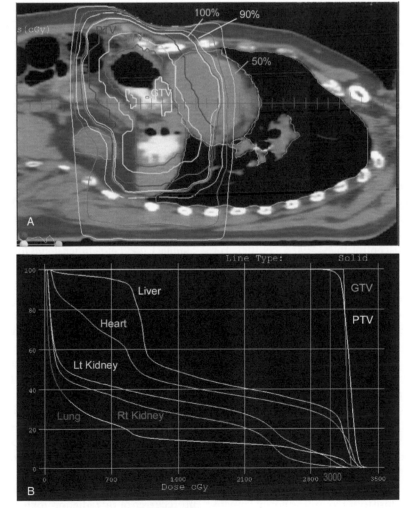

Figure 10.5 Radiation treatment planning (A). Isodose plan, sagittal view (B) DVHs.

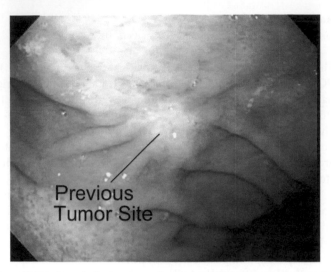

Figure 10.6 Endoscopic disappearance of a gastric MALT lymphoma after radiation therapy.

on the extent of disease and nodal status, and if after surgery, the surgeon's input, including surgical findings, margins and surgical clips. In addition to GTV, CTV and PTV, critical organs like the kidneys, liver, heart and spinal cord should be delineated, spared and monitored. Movements of the stomach must be accounted for at the time of simulation and planning. Patients should be simulated in empty stomach to minimize variation due to gastric content. With the availability of 4D-CT data to analyze intrafraction motion, organ motion can be incorporated in treatment planning and the CTVs at various phases of respiration are fused to form an internal target volume (ITV), which accounts for target motion due to breathing. In addition to anti-emetics, the patient should be fasting the morning of treatment to maintain empty stomach consistency and avoid vomiting and aspiration during treatment.

Although therapeutic doses of radiation for PGL have not been uniformly established, PGL is generally quite radiosensitive and responsive to low doses of radiation. The effective radiation dose range for microscopic, subclinical or small volume gastric MALT lymphoma is approximately 25–30 Gy at 1.5–1.8 Gy per daily fraction with overall long-term control rates >90% [99,108]. For localized gross disease, modest doses of radiation, in the range of 30–36 Gy, have been commonly used with similarly excellent local control [76,97]. As some studies have shown increased local recurrence with <30 Gy, higher doses, ≥40 Gy, have also been used with consistent long-term local control, even if treated with radiation alone [81,109–111].

Three-dimensional Conformal Radiation Therapy, Intensity-modulated Radiation Therapy and Image-guided Radiation Therapy

With continued advances in imaging technology and complex computer planning systems, most patients are currently treated with three-dimensional conformal radiation therapy (3D-CRT), which involves using multiple beams with custom blocks. 3D-CRT markedly enhances accuracy in targeting the tumor, while selectively decreasing the radiation dose to surrounding normal organs and tissues. Conventional treatment method using two opposed AP/PA fields to cover the PTV may often inadvertently lead to surpassing the kidney tolerance. Compared with conventional treatment plans, 3D-CRT plans have demonstrated improved CTV coverage and better normal tissue sparing, especially the liver, kidneys and spinal cord, in treating gastric tumors [112]. The addition of IMRT and IGRT have further customized individual treatment with greater precision and confidence. Although the dose used in PGL is relatively low, the kidney's tolerance can be exceeded, leading to renal atrophy, hypertension or dialysis. IMRT helps spare the kidneys, especially the left kidney, spinal cord and liver that are in close proximity with the target volume.

To evaluate the different treatment planning alternatives, Biancia et al. [113] compared conventional AP/PA and 3D-CRT plans in 15 patients with lymphoma of the stomach. For patients with anatomy having no overlap between PTV and kidneys, there was essentially no benefit from using 3D-CRT over AP/PA. However, for patients with PTVs in close proximity to or overlapping the kidneys, the 4-field 3D-CRT plans were superior with significant reduction of kidney dose. The use of IMRT led to a further reduction in kidney and liver doses in some selected patients.

At the University of Texas Health Science Center in San Antonio, we employ static or dynamic IMRT or TomoTherapy IGRT in the treatment of gastric lymphoma tumors. Four-dimensional (4D) CT is performed to obtain target motion data set to be incorporated into our treatment planning. The combined volume of CTVs obtained at multiple CT phases defines the ITV. Depending on the stage of disease, simultaneous integrated boost technique may be utilized to deliver 25 Gy to PTV and 30 Gy to CTV at 1.5–1.8 Gy daily fraction for gastric MALT lymphoma, with hot spots preferentially over the GTV. For DLBCL, a dose of 30–40 is used. The kidneys and liver are restricted to receive less than 20 and 30 Gy, respectively. Bulky disease may receive a boost of 6–10 Gy to GTV. Usual transient nausea is expected during treatment and can be easily managed with anti-emetics. Adverse toxicity is generally low if proper techniques, planning and doses are used. The rate of hemorrhage or perforation after non-surgical treatment, chemotherapy or chemotherapy and radiation therapy is <5%, typically in patients whose disease is ulcerative, infiltrative and transmural at presentation [105,114].

Sample Case: Four-dimensional Intensity-modulated Radiation Therapy

A 76-year–old Caucasian female presented with several months' history of epigastric pain and weight loss. Her workup led to an endoscopy and biopsies that showed histologic features consistent with low-grade, CD20+, gastric MALT lymphoma not associated with *H. pylori* infection. Fig. 10.1 shows the lesion on endoscopy. Her metastatic workup was negative for distant disease. A CT showed an area of thickened gastric wall (Fig. 10.1). PET and PET/CT confirmed the only site of disease within the fundus (Fig. 10.3). She was stage IE. Primary radiation therapy, static multifield, 4D-IMRT was then utilized. As her disease was small and low-grade, a total dose of 30.6 Gy was delivered to PTV and ITV. Fig. 10.5 illustrates the surrounding anatomical structures and target volumes, isodose plan and DVHs. Her last follow-up at 8 months with endoscopic examination and biopsies showed no recurrence or radiation toxicity thus far. Fig. 10.6 shows the endoscopic disappearance of the tumor after treatment.

Conclusion

Accurate diagnosis and proper staging are paramount to define an appropriate therapeutic option and to avoid over- or undertreatment of patients. Although upfront conservative intervention is utilized in most patients with PGL, the role of surgery includes management of gastric perforation, uncontrolled bleeding or obstruction not responsive to medical or radiation therapy. Jejunostomy feeding tube placement may be required in some patients. In rare occasions, gastrectomy is necessary.

Some patients with a low-grade B-cell MALT-type lymphoma with *H. pylori* infection can be cured with antibiotics treatment. Follow-up is critical as recurrence of MALT lymphomas has been seen years after treatment. Follow-up endoscopic examinations and biopsies, if recurrence is suspected, are necessary to confirm the diagnosis. Other patients with stage I and stage II disease without *H. pylori* infection, and those with *H. pylori* infection but refractory to antibiotics may be treated with systemic chemotherapy (R-CHOP) and radiotherapy. Stage III and IV disease should be treated with systemic chemotherapy and involved-field radiation therapy as indicated. Although technologic advances in radiation treatment planning and delivery have revolutionized radiation therapy, translation into improved clinical outcomes is premature. We have to be aware of the potential long-term effects of low-dose radiation exposure to larger volumes of normal tissue and the risk of marginal miss because of the steep dose gradient in highly conformal IMRT. Successful management depends on an intricate balance of various host factors and treatment parameters. Understanding the day-to-day variations in treatment setup and delivery, determination of proper target volumes and margins without missing the tumor, and judicial use of adequate doses without exceeding normal critical organ tolerances are crucial.

Acknowledgement

The authors wish to thank Drs Michael Dullea, Joseph P Pulcini, and Charles R Thomas, Jr. for their contributions and assistance.

REFERENCES

1. P Brandtzaeg, TS Halstensen, K Kett, et al. Immunobiology and immunopathology of human gut mucosa: humoral immunity and intraepithelial lymphocytes. Gastroenterology 97:1562–84, 1989.
2. M Crump, M Gospodarowicz, FA Shepherd. Lymphoma of the gastrointestinal tract. Semin Oncol 26:324–37, 1999.
3. RE Jones, S Willis, DJ Innes, et al. Primary gastric lymphoma: problems in staging and management. Am J Surg 155:118–23, 1988.
4. RC Thirlby. Gastrointestinal lymphoma: a surgical perspective. Oncology (Huntingt) 7:29–32, 1993.
5. RK Severson, S Davis. Increasing incidence of primary gastric lymphoma. Cancer 66:1283–87, 1990.
6. RS Sandler. Has primary gastric lymphoma become more common? J Clin Gastroenterol 6:101–7, 1984.
7. B Jezersek Novakovic, M Vovk, T Juznic Setina. A single-center study of treatment outcomes and survival in patients with primary gastric lymphomas between 1990 and 2003. Ann Hematol 85(12):849–56, 2006.
8. ES Jaffe, NL Harris, H Stein, et al. (eds) World Health Organization classification of tumours: pathology and genetics of tumours of haematopoietic and lymphoid tissues. Lyon: IARC Press; 2001: 10–11.
9. NL Harris, ES Jaffe, J Diebold, et al. World Health Organization classification of neoplastic diseases of the hematopoietic and lymphoid tissues: report of the Clinical Advisory Committee Meeting—Airlie House, Virginia, November 1997. J Clin Oncol 17:3835–49, 1999.
10. N Jaser, A Sivula, K Franssila. Primary gastric non-Hodgkin's lymphoma in Finland, 1972–1977. Clinical presentation and results of treatment. Scand J Gastroenterol 25(10):1052–59, 1990.
11. A Andriani, A Zullo, F Di Raimondo, et al. Clinical and endoscopic presentation of primary gastric lymphoma: a multicentre study. Aliment Pharmacol Therapeut 23(6): 721–26, 2006.
12. K Contreary, FC Nance, WF Becker. Primary lymphoma of the gastrointestinal tract. Ann Surg 191(5):593–98, 1980.
13. M Raderer, S Wohrer, B Streubel, et al. Assessment of disease dissemination in gastric compared with extragastric mucosa-associated lymphoid tissue lymphoma using extensive staging: a single-center experience J Clin Oncol 24(19):3136–41, 2006.
14. T Suzuki, K Matsuo, H Ito, et al. A past history of gastric ulcers and Helicobacter pylori infection increase the risk of gastric malignant lymphoma. Carcinogenesis. 27(7):1391–97, 2006.
15. C Thorburn, L Rodriguez, J Parsonnet. Epidemiology of gastric non-Hodgkin's lymphoma patients: parallels with Helicobacter pylori. Helicobacter 1(2):75–78, 1996.
16. PF Ferrucci, E Zucca. Primary gastric lymphoma pathogenesis and treatment: what has changed over the past 10 years? Br J Haematol 136(4):521–38, 2007.
17. WS Xu, FC Ho, J Ho, et al. Pathogenesis of gastric lymphoma: the enigma in Hong Kong. Ann Oncol 8(Suppl 2):41–44, 1997.
18. C Portal-Celhay, GI Perez-Perez. Immune responses to Helicobacter pylori colonization: mechanisms and clinical outcomes. Clin Sci (Lond) 110(3):305–14, 2006.
19. M Szczepanik. Interplay between Helicobacter pylori and the immune system. Clinical implications. J Physiol Pharmacol 57(Suppl 3):15–27, 2006.
20. S Wohrer, M Troch, B Streubel, et al. MALT lymphoma in patients with autoimmune diseases: a comparative analysis of characteristics and clinical course. Leukemia 21(8):1812–18, 2007.
21. F Parente, G Rizzardini, M Cernuschi, et al. Non-Hodgkin's lymphoma and AIDS: frequency of gastrointestinal involvement in a large Italian series. Scand J Gastroenterol 28:315–18, 1993.
22. JB Danzig, LJ Brandt, JF Reinus, et al. Gastrointestinal malignancy in patients with AIDS. Am J Gastroenterol 86:715–18, 1991.
23. MS Cappell, N Botros. Predominantly gastrointestinal symptoms and signs in 11 consecutive AIDS patients with gastrointestinal lymphoma: a multicenter, multiyear study including 763 HIV-seropositive patients. Am J Gastroenterol 89:545–49, 1994.

24. J Rodriguez-Sanjuan, A Naranjo, S Echevarria, et al. Primary gastric lymphoma in an HIV-infected patient. J Acquir Immune Defic Syndr Hum Retrovirol 13(5):467–68, 1996.

25. EW Nacoulma, AK Serme, JH Patte, et al. Primary gastric lymphoma complicating HIV infection. Med Trop (Mars) 67(1):61–64, 2007.

26. KR Imrie, CA Sawka, G Kutas, et al. HIV-associated lymphoma of the gastrointestinal tract: the University of Toronto AIDS-Lymphoma Study Group experience. Leuk Lymphoma 16(3–4):343–49, 1995.

27. W Heise, K Arasteh, P Mostertz, et al. Malignant gastro-intestinal lymphomas in patients with AIDS. Digestion 58(3):218–24, 1997.

28. H Inagaki. Mucosa-associated lymphoid tissue lymphoma: molecular pathogenesis and clinicopathological significance. Pathol Int 57(8):474–84, 2007.

29. BS Kahl. Update: gastric MALT lymphoma. Curr Opin Oncol 15(5):347–52, 2003.

30. N Fukuhara, T Nakamura, M Nakagawa, et al. Chromosomal imbalances are associated with outcome of Helicobacter pylori eradication in t(11;18)(q21;q21) negative gastric mucosa-associated lymphoid tissue lymphomas. Genes Chrom Cancer 46(8):784–90, 2007.

31. P Farinha, RD Gascoyne. Molecular pathogenesis of mucosa-associated lymphoid tissue lymphoma. J Clin Oncol 23(26):6370–78, 2005.

32. S Nakamura, S Nakamura, T Matsumoto, et al. Overexpression of caspase recruitment domain (CARD) membrane-associated guanylate kinase 1 (CARMA1) and CARD9 in primary gastric B-cell lymphoma. Cancer 104(9):1885–93, 2005.

33. JO Armitage, DD Weisenburger. New approach to classifying non-Hodgkin's lymphomas: clinical features of the major histologic subtypes. Non-Hodgkin's Lymphoma Classification Project. J Clin Oncol 16:2780–95, 1998.

34. C Thieblemont, Y Bastion, F Berger, et al. Mucosa-associated lymphoid tissue gastrointestinal, and nongastrointestinal lymphoma behavior. Analysis of 108 patients. J Clin Oncol 15:1624–30, 1997.

35. SB Cogliatti, U Schmid, U Schumacher, et al. Primary B-cell gastric lymphoma: a clinicopathological study of 145 patients. Gastroenterology 101(5):1159–70, 1991.

36. PG Gobbi, P Dionigi, F Barbieri, et al. The role of surgery in the multimodal treatment of primary gastric non-Hodgkin's lymphomas: a report of 76 cases and review of the literature. Cancer 65:2528–36, 1990.

37. DN Weingrad, JJ Decosse, P Sherlock, et al. Primary gastrointestinal lymphoma: a 30-year review. Cancer 1982; 49: 1258–65.

38. AM Al-Akwaa, N Siddiqui, IA Al-Mofleh. Primary gastric lymphoma. J World Gastroenterol 10(1):5–11, 2004.

39. IMP Dawson, JS Cornes, BC Morrison. Primary malignant lymphoid tumours of the intestinal tract. Br J Surg 49:80–89, 1961.

40. S Taban, N Tudose. Histologic criteria for the diagnosis of gastric low-grade malt lymphoma. Rom J Morphol Embryol 43(3–4):193–203, 1997.

41. W Zhang, J Garces, HY Dong. Detection of the t(11;18) API2/MALT1 translocation associated with gastric MALT lymphoma in routine formalin-fixed, paraffin-embedded small endoscopic biopsy specimens by robust real-time RT-PCR. Am J Clin Pathol 126(6):931–40, 2006.

42. D Cunningham, T Hickish, RD Rosin, et al. Polymerase chain reaction for detection of dissemination in gastric lymphoma. Lancet 1:695–97, 1989.

43. K Gossios, P Katsimbri, E Tsianos. CT features of gastric lymphoma. Eur Radiol 10(3):425–30, 2000.

44. J Thiele, JP Schneider, F Schmidt, et al. Radiologic imaging of MALT lymphoma (comparison between stomach roentgen image, computerized tomography and magnetic resonance tomography). Aktuelle Radiol 7(6):324–27, 1997.

45. G Caletti, A Ferrari, E Brocchi, et al. Accuracy of endoscopic ultrasonography in the diagnosis and staging of gastric cancer and lymphoma. Surgery 113:14–27, 1993.

46. L Palazzo, G Roseau, A Ruskone-Fourmestraux, et al. Endoscopic ultrasonography in the local staging of primary gastric lymphoma. Endoscopy 25(8):502–8, 1993.

47. V Ambrosini, D Rubello, P Castellucci, et al. Diagnostic role of ^{18}F-FDG PET in gastric MALT lymphoma. Nucl Med Rev Cent East Eur 9(1):37–40, 2006.

48. S Phongkitkarun, V Varavithya, T Kazama, et al. Lymphomatous involvement of gastrointestinal tract: evaluation by positron emission tomography with (18)F-fluorodeoxyglucose. J World Gastroenterol 11(46):7284–89, 2005.

49. T Nihashi, K Hayasaka, T Itou, et al. Findings of fluorine-18-FDG PET in extranodal origin lymphoma—in three cases of diffuse large B cell type lymphoma. Ann Nucl Med 20(10):689–93, 2006.

50. LS Freudenberg, G Antoch, P Schutt, et al. FDG-PET/CT in re-staging of patients with lymphoma. Eur J Nucl Med Mol Imag 31(3):325–29, 2004.

51. L Radan, D Fischer, N Haim, et al. FDG-PET/CT patterns of primary gastric lymphoma. J Nucl Med 48(S2):147P, 2007.

52. C Perry, Y Herishanu, U Metzer, et al. Diagnostic accuracy of PET/CT in patients with extranodal marginal zone MALT lymphoma. J Eur Haematol 79(3):205–9, 2007.

53. SH Sigal, SH Saul, HE Auerbach, et al. Gastric small lymphocytic proliferation with immunoglobulin gene rearrangement in pseudolymphoma versus lymphoma. Gastroenterology 97:195–201, 1989.

54. M Guindi. Role of Helicobacter pylori in the pathogenesis of gastric carcinoma and progression of lymphoid nodules to lymphoma. Can J Gastroenterol 13(3):224–27, 1999.

55. W Fischbach. Primary gastric lymphoma of MALT: considerations of pathogenesis, diagnosis and therapy. Can J Gastroenterol 14(Suppl D):44D–50D, 2000.

56. AC Wotherspoon, C Doglioni, PG Isaacson. Low-grade gastric B-cell lymphoma of mucosa-associated lymphoid tissue (MALT): a multifocal disease. Histopathology 20:29–34, 1992.

57. NL Harris, ES Jaffe, J Diebold, et al. The World Health Organization classification of neoplasms of the hematopoietic and lymphoid tissues: report of the Clinical Advisory Committee meeting. Hematol J 1:53–66, 2000.

58. NL Harris, PG Isaacson. What are the criteria for distinguishing MALT from non-MALT lymphoma at extranodal sites? Am J Clin Pathol 111(1 Suppl 1):S126–32, 1999.

59. C Hsu, CL Chen, LT Chen, et al. Comparison of MALT and non-MALT primary large cell lymphoma of the stomach: does histologic evidence of MALT affect chemotherapy response? Cancer 91(1):49–56, 2001.

60. K Musshoff, H Schmidt-Vollmer. Proceedings: prognosis of non-Hodgkin's lymphomas with special emphasis on the staging classification. Cancer Res Clin Oncol 83:323–41, 1975.

61. J Parsonnet, S Hansen, L Rodriguez, et al. Helicobacter pylori infection and gastric lymphoma. N Engl J Med 330:1267–71, 1994.

62. JM Castrillo, C Montalban, V Abraira, et al. Evaluation of the international index in the prognosis of high grade gastric malt lymphoma. Leuk Lymphoma 24(1–2):159–63, 1996.

63. EM Ibrahim, AA Ezzat, MA Raja, et al. Primary gastric non-Hodgkin's lymphoma: clinical features, management, and prognosis of 185 patients with diffuse large B-cell lymphoma. Ann Oncol 10(12):1441–49, 1999.

64. P Koch, F del Valle, WE Berdel, et al. German Multicenter Study Group. Primary gastrointestinal non-Hodgkin's lymphoma: II. Combined surgical and conservative or conservative management only in localized gastric lymphoma—results of the prospective German Multicenter Study GIT NHL 01/92. J Clin Oncol 19(18):3874–83, 2001.

65. H Medina-Franco, SS Germes, CL Maldonado. Prognostic factors in primary gastric lymphoma. Ann Surg Oncol 14(8):2239–45, 2007.

66. YH Park, WS Kim, SM Bang, et al. Prognostic factor analysis and proposed prognostic model for conventional treatment of high-grade primary gastric lymphoma. Eur J Haematol 77(4):304–8, 2006.

67. T Yoshino, S Nakamura, Y Matsuno, et al. Epstein-Barr virus involvement is a predictive factor for the resistance to chemoradiotherapy of gastric diffuse large B-cell lymphoma. Cancer Sci 97(2):163–66, 2006.

68. P Malfertheiner, F Megraud, C O'Morain, et al. European Helicobacter Pylori Study Group (EHPSG). Current concepts in the management of Helicobacter pylori infection—the Maastricht 2-2000 Consensus Report. Aliment Pharmacol Ther 16(2):167–80, 2002.

69. A Morgner, S Miehlke, W Fischbach, et al. Complete remission of primary high-grade B-cell gastric lymphoma after cure of Helicobacter pylori infection. J Clin Oncol 19(7):2041–48, 2001.

70. AC Wotherspoon. A critical review of the effect of Helicobacter pylori eradication on gastric MALT lymphoma. Curr Gastroenterol Rep 2(6):494–98, 2000.

71. E Roggero, E Zucca, G Pinotti, et al. Eradication of HELICOBACTER pylori infection in primary low-grade gastric lymphoma of mucosa-associated lymphoid tissue. Ann Intern Med 122:767–69, 1995.

72. AC Wotherspoon, C Doglioni, TC Diss, et al. Regression of primary low-grade B-cell gastric lymphoma of mucosa-associated lymphoid tissue type after eradication of Helicobacter pylori. Lancet 342:575–77, 1993.

73. WD Chey, BC Wong. Practice Parameters Committee of the American College of Gastroenterology. American College of Gastroenterology guideline on the management of Helicobacter pylori infection. Am J Gastroenterol 102(8):1808–25, 2007.

74. W Fischbach, Goebeler-Kolve, P Starostik, et al. Minimal residual low-grade gastric MALT-type lymphoma after eradication of Helicobacter pylori. Lancet 360(9332):547–48, 2002.

75. T Akamatsu, T Mochizuki, Y Okiyama, et al. Comparison of localized gastric mucosa-associated lymphoid tissue (MALT) lymphoma with and without Helicobacter pylori infection. Helicobacter 11(2):86–95, 2006.

76. M Sugimoto, M Kajimura, N Shirai, et al. Outcome of radiotherapy for gastric mucosa-associated lymphoid tissue lymphoma refractory to Helicobacter pylori eradication therapy. Intern Med 45(6):405–9, 2006.

77. RW Tsang, MK Gospodarowicz. Low-grade non-Hodgkin's lymphomas. Sem Radiat Oncol 17(3):198–205, 2007.

78. S Nakamura, K Akazawa, T Yao, et al. A clinicopathologic study of 233 cases with special reference to evaluation with the MIB-1 index. Cancer 76:1313–24, 1995.

79. R Caronna, M Cardi, M Martelli, et al. Systematic radical gastrectomy and D2 lymphadenectomy in primary gastric B cell lymphoma: impact on diagnosis, classification and long term results. A prospective study. J Chemother 16(Suppl 5):26–29, 2004.

80. G Salles, R Herbrecht, H Tilly, et al. Aggressive primary gastrointestinal lymphomas: review of 91 patients treated with the LNH-84 regimen. Am J Med 90:77–84, 1991.

81. A Aviles, MJ Nambo, N Neri, et al. The role of surgery in primary gastric lymphoma: results of a controlled clinical trial. Ann Surg 240(1):44–50, 2004.

82. A Aviles, N Neri, MJ Nambo, et al. Surgery and chemotherapy versus chemotherapy as treatment of high-grade MALT gastric lymphoma. Med Oncol 23(2):295–300, 2006.

83. S Yoon, DG Coit, CS Portlock, et al. The diminishing role of surgery in the treatment of gastric lymphoma. Ann Surg 240(1):28–37, 2004.

84. M Kochi, M Fujii, N Kanamori, et al. Complete remission by chemotherapy in stage IE-IIE primary gastric lymphoma. Hepato-Gastroenterology 54(76):1285–88, 2007.

85. M Raderer, J Valencak, C Osterreicher, et al. Chemotherapy for the treatment of patients with primary high grade gastric B-cell lymphoma of modified Ann Arbor Stages IE and IIE. Cancer 88(9):1979–85, 2000.

86. M Binn, A Ruskone-Fourmestraux, E Lepage, et al. Surgical resection plus chemotherapy versus chemotherapy alone: comparison of two strategies to treat diffuse large B-cell gastric lymphoma. Ann Oncol 14(12):1751–57, 2003.

87. M Raderer, A Chott, J Drach, et al. Chemotherapy for management of localised high-grade gastric B-cell lymphoma: how much is necessary? Ann Oncol 13(7):1094–98, 2002.

88. AJ Ferreri, S Cordio, M Ponzoni, et al. Non-surgical treatment with primary chemotherapy, with or without radiation therapy, of stage I–II high-grade gastric lymphoma. Leuk Lymphoma 33(5–6):531–41, 1999.

89. N Haim, M Leviov, Y Ben-Arieh, et al. Intermediate and high-grade gastric non-Hodgkin's lymphoma: a prospective study of non-surgical treatment with primary chemotherapy, with or without radiotherapy. Leuk Lymphoma 17(3–4):321–26, 1995.

90. S Ishikura, K Tobinai, A Ohtsu, et al. Japanese multicenter phase II study of CHOP followed by radiotherapy in stage I–II, diffuse large B-cell lymphoma of the stomach. Cancer Sci 96(6):349–52, 2005.

91. YH Park, SH Lee, WS Kim, et al. CHOP followed by involved field radiotherapy for localized primary gastric diffuse large B-cell lymphoma: results of a multi center phase II study and quality of life evaluation. Leuk Lymphoma 47(7):1253–59, 2006.

92. RA Popescu, AC Wotherspoon, D Cunningham, et al. Surgery plus chemotherapy or chemotherapy alone for primary intermediate- and high-grade gastric non-Hodgkin's lymphoma: the Royal Marsden Hospital experience. Eur J Cancer 35(6):928–34, 1999.

93. A Solidoro, C Payet, J Sanchez-Lihon, et al. Gastric lymphomas: chemotherapy as a primary treatment. Semin Surg Oncol 6:218–25, 1990.

94. S Wohrer, A Puspok, J Drach, et al. Rituximab, cyclophosphamide, doxorubicin, vincristine and prednisone (R-CHOP) for treatment of early-stage gastric diffuse large B-cell lymphoma. Ann Oncol 15(7):1086–90, 2004.

95. G Martinelli, D Laszlo, AJ Ferreri, et al. Clinical activity of rituximab in gastric marginal zone non-Hodgkin's lymphoma resistant to or not eligible for anti-Helicobacter pylori therapy. J Clin Oncol 23(9):1979–83, 2005.

96. A Morgner, R Schmelz, C Thiede, et al. Therapy of gastric mucosa associated lymphoid tissue lymphoma. World J Gastroenterol 13(26):3554–66, 2007.

97. J Yahalom, C Portlock, M Gonzales, et al. H. plyori-independent MALT lymphoma of the stomach: excellent outcome with radiation alone. Blood 100:160a (abstr), 2002.

98. NR Schechter, J Yahalom. Low-grade MALT lymphoma of the stomach: a review of treatment options. Int J Radiat Oncol Biol Phys 46:1093–1103, 2000.

99. ML Lin, A Wirth, M Chao, et al. Radiotherapy for low-grade gastric marginal zone lymphoma: a retrospective study. Intern Med J 37(3):172–80, 2007.

100. RW Tsang, MK Gospodarowicz, M Pintilie, et al. Localized mucosa-associated lymphoid tissue lymphoma treated with radiation therapy has excellent clinical outcome. J Clin Oncol 21:4157–64, 2003.

101. J Yahalom, NR Schechter, M Gonzales. Effective treatment of MALT lymphoma of the stomach with radiation alone (Abstr.). Ann Oncol 10:135, 1999.

102. T Sano. Treatment of primary gastric lymphoma: experience in the National Cancer Center Hospital, Tokyo. Recent Results Cancer Res 156:104–7, 2000.

103. DA Haber. MRJ: primary gastrointestinal lymphoma. Semin Oncol 15:154–69, 1988.

104. MM Law, SB Williams, JH Wong. Role of surgery in the management of primary lymphoma of the gastrointestinal tract. J Surg Oncol 61:199–204, 1996.

105. B Mittal, TH Wasserman, RC Griffith. Non-Hodgkin's lymphoma of the stomach. J Am Gastroenterol 78(12):780–87, 1983.

106. P Koch, F del Valle, WE Berdel, et al. German Multicenter Study Group. Primary gastrointestinal non-Hodgkin's lymphoma: I. Anatomic and histologic distribution, clinical features, and survival data of 371 patients registered in the German Multicenter Study GIT NHL 01/92. J Clin Oncol 19(18):3861–73, 2001.

107. P Koch, A Probst, WE Berdel, et al. Treatment results in localized primary gastric lymphoma: data of patients registered within the German multicenter study (GIT NHL 02/96). J Clin Oncol 23(28):7050–59, 2005.

108. RW Tsang, MK Gospodarowicz, M Pintilie, et al. Stage I and II MALT lymphoma: results of treatment with radiotherapy. J Int Radiat Oncol Biol Phys 50(5):1258–64, 2001.

109. N Schechter, CS Portlock, J Yahalom. Treatment of mucosa-associated lymphoid tissue lymphoma of the stomach with radiation alone. J Clin Oncol 16(5):1916–21, 1998.

110. CY Fung, ML Grossbard, RM Linggood, et al. Mucosa-associated lymphoid tissue lymphoma of the stomach: long term outcome after local treatment. Cancer 85(1):9–17, 1999.

111. DS Shimm, DE Dosoretz, T Anderson, et al. Primary gastric lymphoma. An analysis with emphasis on prognostic factors and radiation therapy. Cancer 52(11):2044–48, 1983.

112. S Garcia, S Krishnan, N Tucker, et al. Dosimetric comparison of conventional AP-PA plus oblique, 3D, coplanar IMRT, and non-coplanar IMRT techniques in the treatment of gastric lymphoma. Int J Radiat Oncol Biol Phys 66(3):S507, 2006.

113. C Della Biancia, M Hunt, E Furhang, et al. Radiation treatment planning techniques for lymphoma of the stomach. J Int Radiat Oncol Biol Phys 62(3):745–51, 2005.

114. N Maisey, A Norman, Y Prior, et al. Chemotherapy for primary gastric lymphoma: does in-patient observation prevent complications? Clin Oncol (Royal Col Radiol) 16(1):48–52, 2004.

115. C Thieblemont, C Dumontet, F Bouafia, et al. Outcome in relation to treatment modalities in 48 patients with localized gastric MALT lymphoma: a retrospective study of patients treated during 1976–2001. Leuk Lymphoma 44(2):257–62, 2003.

116. RK Valicenti, TH Wasserman, NA Kucik. Analysis of prognostic factors in localized gastric lymphoma: the importance of bulk of disease. Int J Radiat Oncol Biol Phys 27(3):591–98, 1993.

117. W Fischbach, B Dragosics, ME Kolve-Goebeler, et al. Primary gastric B-cell lymphoma: results of a prospective multicenter study. The German-Austrian Gastrointestinal Lymphoma Study Group. Gastroenterology 119(5):1191–1202 (erratum appears in Gastroenterology 2000; 119(6):1809), 2000.

Index

T - #0591 - 071024 - C96 - 279/216/5 - PB - 9780367384487 - Gloss Lamination